COVID-19:
Because What You Don't Know Will Kill You

Alan H.B. Wu, Ph.D.

Covid-19! Because what you don't know will kill you contains fictitious characters, events, and places. Any resemblance to actual persons, living or dead, business establishments, events, or locales is entirely coincidental. The science described in these stories, however, is factual.

ISBN-13: 978-0-9973686-8-0
eBook ISBN: 978-0-9973686-9-7

Dedication
This book is dedicated to my wife my lifelong companion, and my children, especially Kimberly, who have supported my work throughout the years.

Acknowledgements
I thank Dr. Valerie Ng, Chief of Staff at Highland Hospital, Oakland CA, and Ms. Cassandra Yun for their critical review and editing of the content.

Table of Contents

Prologue

Not since the outbreak of the Second World War has any single event caused so much suffering as the COVID-19 pandemic. In December 2019, the outbreak of SARS-CoV-2 changed the world in ways that were unimaginable in the months prior to the virus' existence. In early July of 2020, the number of deaths worldwide caused by COVID-19 infection exceeded the total suffered by World War II. To find an event equally tragic, one would have to go back to the 6th and 7th Centuries AD where an estimated 50 million people died of the bubonic plague.

In 2014, I took on the mission to educate the general public on the value of clinical laboratory testing through the authorship and release of five paperback and electronic books. The stories are based on real cases where clinical laboratory testing was instrumental in solving important medical questions, or where neglect or misuse of lab results caused medical errors. In writing these stories, I hoped to inspire the public to have a greater awareness of the value of clinical laboratory science and for everyone to take a more active role in the medical decisions made on them and their loved ones. All of these stories were written from my perspective as a clinical laboratory director, drawing from my nearly 40 years of experience on the job. They provide a "behind the scenes" view of the profession. Some of these books have been translated into Italian, simplified and traditional Chinese, and Korean

My first book, *Toxicology! Because What You Don't Know Can Kill You*, highlights drug testing and is the most popular of my books. Readers are interested in crime and punishment, although not necessarily in a legal sense, but on the toll drug abuse takes on human life. The book has been translated into Italian and Korean. In this latest edition, I have added two new stories, *The Hall of Flame*, and *Blitz*, written after the book's initial release.

The book, *Hidden Assassin: When Clinical Lab Tests Go Awry*, describes stories that center around specialized clinical chemistry and molecular diagnostics. These are "mainstream" tests that are done in every hospital in the world today and affects every human on the planet. This book has been translated into Italian and Chinese (both traditional and simplified, and soon to be Spanish).

My third book is *Microbiology! Because What You Don't Know Will Kill You*, written before the COVID-19 pandemic. I describe stories about microbiologic infections and the role of the clinical laboratory. There were no stories about coronavirus, even though there was an outbreak in China in 2003. But then in late 2019, COVID-19 hit Wuhan and soon it would spread to the rest of the world.

An important aspect to the spread of this virus has been the lack of testing availability. Individuals who are free from symptoms can unknowingly spread this virus to others. The inability of the lab to meet medical demands has shown to everyone now why testing is so important and why the clinical laboratory should not be the place to cut costs. Prior to COVID-19, reimbursements were reduced by the government for laboratory testing leading to supply shortages that can be directly linked to deaths.

I wrote this book because of the dramatic events that took place in 2020. In the first part of my book, I have assembled information on what the virus is, how it is transmitted to humans, how individuals can be treated, and the importance of human immunity against the virus. As with my other books, this is followed by stories of people, some real, some fictionalized.

As a clinical laboratory scientist at a major academic medical center, I get questions from physicians and other healthcare workers regarding the virology of Severe Acute Respiratory Syndrome Coronavirus 2 (SARS-CoV-2), the medical consequences of an infection, and the science behind testing of human samples. While I am not a microbiologist by training or profession, when it comes to managing COVID-19 infections, all of us in the clinical lab despite our background, have quickly been brought up to speed with the science in order to do our part in caring for patients and reducing spread of the disease. I am a trained "translational scientist" meaning that I can read and understand the basic scientific literature and understand how this knowledge can be applied to affect medical practices. I have published nearly 500 peer-reviewed publications, I am peer reviewer for dozens of submitted manuscripts (including many on COVID-19), and Editor-in-Chief for two scientific journals. My research involves conducting clinical trials on novel diagnostic and prognostic tests prior to their use in medical practices. I am therefore qualified to evaluate science and medicine. In order to maintain my professional credibility, it is essential that I report my findings without bias or meeting a political agenda.

As a clinical laboratory director, the implementation of many of these discoveries into routine medical practice is my job. During the pandemic, I have read hundreds of papers, and given talks to our staff, physicians, and national and international meetings to the medical and scientific communities. Moreover, I have fielded questions posed by local and national print media and news programs that reach the lay audience.

In writing this book, I have "borrowed" stories from three of my prior books and have written sequel stories that involves COVID-19. It was necessary to include these older stories ("Mysophobia," "Urine Luck," "Accident Aftermath," "Mind Portal: How it Began," and "Ashwood") for the reader to understand the context of these new stories ("The Hand Sanitizer," and "The Parade," respectively).

A.H.B. Wu, Palo Alto, CA. March, 2021.

SARS-CoV-2: Transmission

****

"Coronavirus" (CoV) refers to a family of viruses that have a similar structure, including the presence of spikes on the surface of the cell. There are several coronaviruses that have been described through history. The term SARS refers to Severe Acute Respiratory Syndrome. SARS-CoV refers to the original SARS infection that occurred in China in 2003. The SARS-CoV-2 refers to the virus that started in Wuhan in December of 2019. The term, "COVID-19" refers to the 2019 COrona VIrus Disease.

Science versus political gain was a major theme in the U.S. 2020 Presidential Elections. Both sides could be accused of bending the truth to meet their political need. Now that the 2020 elections have ended and a new Administration has been elected, it is time to review what we know about the virus that causes COVID-19 and testing for it, without political motivation. In addressing these issues, one must conduct a critical review of the available evidence published in scientific and medical journals. Particularly important is an assessment of the methodology used, results obtained, and conclusions rendered by the authors. In compiling this summary, I have sought out and cited studies conducted by accomplished scientists and physicians and published in the most reputable journals in the world. Acceptance into this literature requires peer review. Often, there are several rounds of submissions and revisions between the reviewers and authors. Physicians rely on reports from these journals to make important medical decisions regarding the health and wellbeing of their patients, which is the only agenda.

For the lay public, I have listed some of the source documents that I have relied upon to render my conclusions. The review of the original data will enable a motivated reader to formulate their own opinions. This is the accepted manner by which dissemination of scientific information is performed. As part of the scientific process, one should not accept the opinion of one author or group as necessarily being the truth. It is important that these reports be vetted for relevance, bias, and potential agenda.

This is very much unlike the manner by which information is transmitted to the lay media, where there is no systematic peer review. Reporters release stories based on their sources, with readers relying on a reporter's reputation and those of the media outlet, to ensure that the information presented is factual. Truth in reporting was not challenged in the pre-internet era. The term "fake news" might only have been used in a comedy sketch. Today, misinformation and misdirection are major political tools. Popular internet websites have become the conduit of fake news, as social networks are not able to verify or take responsibility for the content it hosts.

What follows are referenced discussions on important COVID-19 topics. This is important because "What you don't know will kill you."

COVID-19 virus and viral proteins

The coronavirus is spherical in shape with spikes scattered throughout the surface of the virus (see our book cover!) Some believe that the virus was name due to their resemblance of spikes on a crown. The name, however, comes from images from an electron microscope, where the protrusions more closely resemble a halo or the corona of the sun.

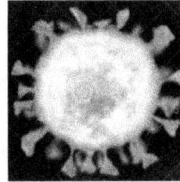

The coronavirus spikes play a key functional role as they are used by the virus to gain entry into a host cell. Acting like a door "key," these spikes binds to a specific receptor of a cell to gain entry, just as a key opens a lock. Once inside, the virus hijacks the cell's adopted home, and it uses the cell's protein manufacturing facility to reproduce itself rather than the cell's normal protein-producing function. Imagine a guest comes to your home, takes over the kitchen, and makes food that is nourishing for the guest so they can multiply, while being poisonous to the host such that everybody in the family dies and the guests survive? The cell dies, and the newly created copies of the virus are then released into the body to infect new cells. Because this amplification cycle takes time, all infectious diseases have an "incubation" phase, meaning that an individual is not symptomatic or does not have high bacterial or viral counts in their bodies for a few days. In addition to the spike protein, coronavirus has structural proteins that make up its shell to contain its nuclear material, and functional proteins that help direct its reproduction. Contained with the spike's protein sequence is the receptor binding domain (RBD). As the name implies, the RBD is the specific part of the spike protein that is able to bind to the host receptor. For human infections, the angiotensin converting enzyme-2 (ACE2) receptor is that part of the cell that is found in abundant quantities within pneumocytes (pulmonary cells). and explains why SARS-CoV-2 is a respiratory virus.

Where does it come from?

Scientists use genetic sequence data to hypothesize on the origin of this virus. Based on a 96% viral nucleic acid sequence similarity, some have opined that SARS-CoV-2 originated through the consumption of horseshoe bat meat (Touati et al.). Others during the early stages of the pandemic suggested there is no direct transmission from bats and that an intermediate host is required. The pangolin (scaly anteater found in Asia and Africa) has been suggested to be the culprit. More recent studies have exonerated this animal as a vector for transmission of the virus (Frutos et al.). Before then, this theory led to the unnecessary killing of some of these innocent animals, in an attempt to curb the pandemic. It

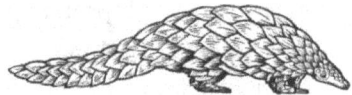

may be a few more years, if ever, before the exact origin of this killer virus is known.

While it is clear that the COVID-19 outbreak began in December 2019 in Wuhan China, what is unknown is how SARS-CoV-2 was created. Conspiracy theorists believe the virus was artificially mutated by geneticists in hopes of developing vaccines to other viruses such as HIV. A dire and more disturbing hypothesis is that this work was in an attempt to develop a more powerful biological weapon. Such a sinister objective has been the topic of science fiction cinema. It is hard to fathom that intelligent civilizations and governments would have this as an objective. If it was the purpose, to exterminate millions of humans on the planet, the program has succeeded beyond anybody's wildest nightmare. At this date, there is no scientific evidence that this virus was created artificially. There are no documents that show this objective or scientific reports describing how this work could be accomplished. There is also no paper trail regarding the funding that it would require to undertake such a mission. The best knowledge we have today, is that this virus was mutated naturally from previous coronaviruses that has been known for decades.

The airborne route of COVID-19 infection

The route of transmission for a respiratory virus is direct contact (e.g., kissing), secondary direct contact (e.g., hand shaking followed by touching the contaminated mouth, nose, or other mucous membranes), and airborne (e.g., inhalation of droplets from an infected individual who has coughed, sneezed or expelled virus while talking).

A cough produces an estimated 3,000 droplets while a sneeze can release 10 times that amount. As one would expect, the distance traveled by expelled droplets is further for sneezes than coughs. Fortunately, patients with COVID-19 infections typically suffer from repeated coughs and not sneezes. Most of the time, COVID-19 infected individuals have dry coughs, i.e., there is no mucous or phlegm released at the same time. Airborne transmission of SARS-CoV-2 occurs through the exposure of droplets from the host. The size of the droplets formed depends on their origin.

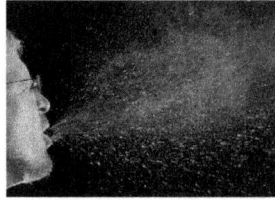

The largest droplets (100 μm) come from the mouth. Given their size, these expelled droplets that occur through talking flow to the ground by gravity and do not travel very far from the source. Unless someone is very near the person talking, e.g., one foot or less, this is not a frequent source of viral transmissions. People who engage in heated arguments are particularly vulnerable if one of them is infected with COVID-19. Individuals who give lectures or speeches, such as professors and especially politicians have the potential to infect more individuals because they talk louder, for longer periods of time, and often more vigorously than during common conversation (now have a medical reason for disliking loud mouths). Using laser light scattering methods,

Stadnytskyi et al. showed that several thousands of droplets are formed per second. The smallest droplets can remain in a stagnant air environment for 8-14 minutes. The audience should stand further away from the orator. During the U.S. vice presidential debate in 2020, a plexiglass screen was interspersed between the candidates. As discussed in the next section, plastic barriers may not be the best choice of materials to use. When a talk has ended, the space around the speaker should be thoroughly disinfected by workers who themselves must be protected by donning personal protective equipment.

Coughs and sneezes are a major source of COVID-19 transmission. A cough produces smaller droplets ranging from 1-100 μm. They are expelled in the form of a aerosols which can travel 6-20 feet. It has been estimated that 100 μm droplets take 10 seconds to reach the ground where as 10 μm droplets can linger for 17 minutes or more (Dhand et al., Dorelalen et al.). Smaller droplets can linger for much longer. Fortunately, most droplets from an infected patient do not contain any virion, and the probability of a 10 μm droplet containing SARS-CoV-2 may be less than 1%. Larger droplets have a proportionally higher likelihood of containing a viral particle. The surrounding air environment is an important factor. With strong ventilation or wind in the case of outdoors, droplets are carried further away from the source. At the same time, good air flow disperses aerosols and droplets thereby diluting the density of virus for a given volume of gas, making it less infectious. As the nation slowly opened up after the initial lock down, it was medically acceptable to re-open parks and beaches for the activities of normal daily living, with a recommendation of social distancing, and permit outdoor dining and participation in individual leisure sports such as golf and surfing.

Stability of SARS-CoV-2 on various surfaces

COVID-19 infections can also occur if droplets settle onto surfaces and an individual first touches those surfaces and

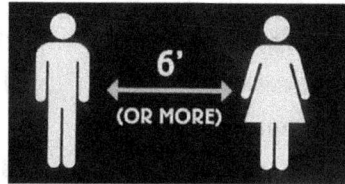

then touches their mouth, nose, or eyes. Therefore, the stability of SARS-CoV-2 on various surfaces become an important variable and determinant to our daily lives. Several studies have examined the viability of the virus on various surfaces. These are not easy or fun experiments to perform. Researchers use live and highly infectious viruses in these studies, and there is no effective treatment or vaccine available when the studies are conducted. One study examined stability on plastic, stainless steel, copper and cardboard (Doremalen et al.). Another examined swine skin, currency, and clothing. Combining the two studies following room temperature storage, the virus broke down within 4 hours when placed on clothing, 8 hours on copper and circulating currency, 24 hours on cardboard, 48 hours on steel, 72 hours on plastic, and 96 hours on skin. Increasing temperatures degrade the virus faster, therefore there is no transmission from cooked food. Studies have shown that the virus has a half-life of under 1 minute when heated at 70 °C when the dish is uncovered but is more stable when covered (Gamble). Heating food with a microwave oven will also be effective if put on high power.

Human skin on a live person is closer to body temperature, where the virus is degraded after 8 hours. Active movement of fingers and contact with other materials during the course of daily activity may expel the virus from the skin and decrease its infectivity. Lower temperatures, however, stabilize the virus. Nevertheless, these studies suggest that virus transmission is possible through surface contact. An infection does require exposure to the individual's nose, mouth or skin that that has an open wound.

The outdoor exposure has a significant effect on the spread and stability of SARS-CoV-2. Any degree of wind flow will disperse and dilute infected droplets. Ultraviolet rays generated from the sun can greatly inactivate the virus. It has been known for many years that UV light below 315 nm (UVB and UVC) are particularly effective in inactivating bacteria and viruses. These rays also produce tanning of the skin and melanomas. UV light is strongest when the sun is directly overhead, i.e., the summer months, near the equator, and at noon time. Specific SARS-CoV-2 studies have shown that the stability of the virus can be less than 5 minutes under direct exposure to UV light (Hermann et al.). This is why local health departments have allowed outdoor activities such as dining, if individuals can maintain social distancing.

The mechanism for the differences in SARS-CoV-2 survival on different surfaces was studied by Harbout et al. He suggested that materials that absorbs water such as clothing and paper dries the droplet rending it inactive. Plastic and steel are not able to wick water away. Copper being non-porous is an exception and may relate to the metal's oxidant activity. With this knowledge, one might expect an interest in installing copper doorknobs. What hasn't been studied is how sticky the virus is when the surfaces are moved and handled. In an extreme case, will a tennis ball that travels 100 miles per hour after being struck retain coronavirus on its surface? In the absence of these answers, the recommendations made by all world and national health bodies for frequent handwashing is very prudent.

Disinfectants

There has been little debate regarding the choice of disinfectants. Products containing bleach and alcohol are widely used and are effective. Early in the pandemic, there were shortages of hand sanitizers, prompting some manufacturers of alcoholic beverages to switch production of drinks to sanitizers. As a hospital that treats a large homeless population, I received a question about the effect of alcoholism on risk for a COVID-19 infection. There are three factors that suggest that drinking could be protective: 1) alcohol is excreted in the breath after consumption, 2) alcohol is the active ingredient in disinfectants, and 3) SARS-CoV-2 is transmitted through inhalation. We conducted a study of excessive alcohol drinking by alcoholics. Among emergency department admissions at our hospital, we determined if the frequency of a COVID-19 infection was lower in individuals with high concentrations of alcohol in their blood than individuals who had a negative alcohol result. In the end, we found no difference in the incidence of COVID infection. Extreme ethanol consumption is not protective. The effective alcohol concentration needed in hand sanitizing and disinfectant products is much higher than what can be produced in blood after excessive intake (Lebin et al.). Intoxication may provide only a mental escape from the risk of an infection. Likewise, oral ingestion of disinfectants, particularly ammonia or chlorine-based solutions or high concentrations of hydrogen peroxide is especially hazardous to delicate gastrointestinal tissues such as the esophagus. The suggestion of taking Chlorox baths by Cristina Cuomo, wife of CNN News anchor Chris Cuomo and sister-in-law to the governor of New York, is without scientific basis.

The mask controversy

The 2020 Presidential election polarized the nation in unprecedented ways. Democrats pushed for wearing masks while Republicans did not support this practice systematically. Scientists have also debated on the importance of wearing masks. Early in the pandemic, both surgical masks and respirators (N95 masks) were in short supply. Most of the masks used in America were made in China, who were sequestering these supplies to handle their own pandemic. The decision to mandate mask wearing was academic: healthcare workers got priority for the precious few that were available. After many months, the shortage of masks, respirators, and other personal protective equipment has now eased. The debate on universal mask usage continues (Greenhalgh et al).

N95 respirators are so named because when properly fitted and worn, it can block the passage of 95% of airborne particles as small as 0.3 microns in size. The objective is to protect the wearer, typically a healthcare worker, from contracting an infection. Some of these respirators have an exhaust valve to facilitate breathing and may be more useful for industrial use. Fitting is more difficult to achieve on individuals with facial hair. Critics of mask and respirator use state that the SARS-CoV-2 virus is less than half that size and therefore these respirators cannot block passage of the virus. However, the virus is expelled into larger droplets which are blocked by the respirators, as it is unlikely that active virus floats freely (i.e., unattached to a droplet) into the atmosphere.

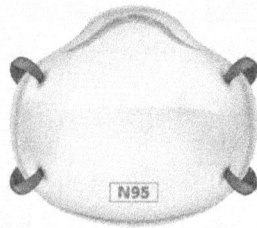

Randomized controlled trials conducted among healthcare workers have demonstrated that wearing surgical masks and N95 respirators can reduce the risks of contracting a respiratory virus. For respiratory infections including influenza as the model, MacIntyre et al. reviewed the literature and reported a 25-60% reduction in infections demonstrating that N95 respirators are effective.

Surgical masks consist of a three-ply polypropylene material designed to capture droplets from an individual who is sneezing or coughs. It is used by individuals to protect a person from infecting others. These masks can also be worn by patients to protect individuals who are caring for them. This is not possible for seriously ill patients in intensive care units, on ventilators or are intubated.

It has been known since the beginning of the COVID-19 pandemic that infected individuals who are asymptomatic can unknowingly spread the virus to others. This can be a source of infection, even from individuals wearing surgical masks. Unlike the N95 respirator, surgical masks are loosely worn with straps that loop around the ears. There is a metal piece at the top of the mask that should be pinched around the nose to provide a tighter seal.

There have been no studies involving use of less expensive surgical or cloth masks, but this is still superior to not wearing any face coverings. In high risk situations, there is merit in double masking for individuals who don't have access to N95 respirators.

The psychological effect of wearing a mask is an important variable in this discussion. In the U.S., mask wearing is associated with villainous behavior, like bank robbers. While there are some heroes who wear masks like Batman, Spiderman, and Zorro, the American culture is largely negative toward masks and will have to be reversed to curb this pandemic (it was unclear why Wonder Woman never needed to hide her identity). Many Asian countries have endorsed mask wearing as an infection control measure for many years. This may be a combination of more respiratory disease outbreaks (e.g., the bird flu), a higher density of the population within their cities, and in some cases, a tighter control of individual freedoms. The reluctance of political leaders to ignore health mandates reflects an attitude of arrogance and does not establish a good image of compliance to the rest of the citizenship. Individuals who wear masks in public are more likely to adhere to personal hygiene practices like hand washing, social distancing, and limiting participation by large gatherings.

References

Dhand R, et al. Coughs and sneezes: their role in transmission of respiratory viral infections, including SARS-CoV-2. Am J Resp Crit Care Med 2020;202:651-9.

Frutos R, et ta. COVID-19: Time to exonerate the pangolin from the transmission of SARS-CoV-2 to humans. Infect Gen Evol 2020; doi.org/10.1016/j.meegid.2020.104493

Gamble A, et al. Heat-treated virus inactivation rate depends strongly on treatment procedure. bioRxiv. 2020;

doi: 10.1101/2020.08.10.242206

Greenhalgh T, et al. Face masks for the public during the covid-19 crisis. BMJ 2020 doi:10.1136/bjm1435

Harbout DE, et al. Modeling the stability of severe acute respiratory syndrome coronavirus 2 (SARS-2-CoV-2) on skin, currency, and clothing. PLOS 2020, doi:org/10.1371/journal.pntd.0008831.

Hermann J, et al. Inactivation times from 290 to 315 nm UVB in sunlight for SARS coronaviruses CoV and CoV-2 using OMI satellite date for the sunlit Earth. Air Qual Atmosph Health 2020; doi.org/10.1007/s11869-020-00927-2.

Lebin J, et al. Chronic alcohol use does not protect against Covid-19 infection. Am J Emerg Med 2020; doi.org/10.1016/j.ajem2020.11.024

MacIntyre CR, et al. Facemasks for the prevention of infections in healthcare and community settings. BMJ 2015;350:h694.

Stadnytskyi V, et al. The airborne lifetime of small speech droplets and their potential importance in SARS-CoV-2 transmission. PNAS 2020;117:11875-7.

Touati R, et al. Comparative genomic signature representations of the emerging COVID-19 coronavirus and other coronaviruses: High identity and possible recombination between bat and pangolin coronaviruses. Gen 2020;42:4189-202.

Dorelalen N, et al. Aerosol and surface stability of SARS-CoV-2 as compared with SARS-CoV1. N Engl J Med

2020 doi:10.1056/NEJM c2004973

Testing for SARS CoV-2

****

The key to controlling the pandemic is testing someone for the presence of the coronavirus. There are many ways to test an individual to see if they have been infected with SARS-CoV-2. Each of these methods have advantages and disadvantages. Some additional details on testing can be found scattered with the stories that follow this introduction. Under pre-pandemic conditions, manufacturers of new medical tests must receive approval by the Food and Drug Administration prior to their release and use by clinical labs. This requires submission of data from clinical trials of several thousand individuals that confirm the medical claims made by the manufacturer of the test instrument or reagent, a process that can take years. For example, if a new test is to be used to diagnose heart failure, a high proportion of heart failure patients should have a positive test result, while a high proportion of patients without heart failure should have a negative result. These studies can cost millions of dollars to a company.

Once tests are approved, the testing itself in is conducted in laboratories certified by the Centers for Medicare and Medicaid. These clinical laboratories are required to follow regulations outlined by the Clinical Laboratory Improvement Amendment (or CLIA), established in 1988. Individuals performing testing within clinical laboratories are termed "Clinical Laboratory Scientists" (or CLS) and are licensed by a state where the laboratory is located, or through national accreditation programs. These individuals are not only trained to perform the test properly, but to spot trouble should the assays produce erroneous results. Licensed laboratory directors and/or pathologists have the responsibility for communicating test results and interpretations to individuals, particularly physicians, who order the test.

The approval process for COVID-19 lab tests was greatly accelerated in an effort to get the important tests needed for diagnosis of the disease and for quarantine decisions. Due to the public health emergency, the FDA recognized that laboratory tests have a significant potential to affect national security or the health of U.S. citizens. They therefore enacted "Emergency Use Authorization" or EUA. This allowed test manufacturers to conduct validation studies on hundreds rather than thousands of subjects in order to receive approval and release of test devices for clinical use within weeks and not years. The first COVID-19 test was the Centers for Disease Control and Prevention's PCR test, approved on February 2, 2020, well before there was widespread infection in the country.

The human specimen of choice for both the viral RNA and proteins is to swab the nasal pharyngeal (NP)

cavity. The long NP swab is inserted deep
into the nasal cavity towards the back of
the throat.   The procedure can be
uncomfortable and painful.   During the
early stages of the pandemic, this was the
preferred sample for diagnostic purposes
because the virus concentration was higher there.

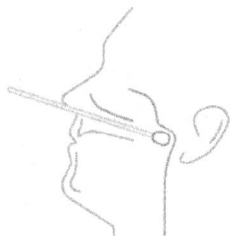

More recently, samples from other more assessable
parts of the head are used including the mid nasal cavity,
throat, and saliva. The sensitivity for viral RNA detection
from these samples was thought to be lower than for an NP
swab, but recent studies have shown that these samples could
be equivalent to an NP swab. For viral antigen testing, the
immunoassay technique is easier and faster than PCR. For
mass screening of the population, these immunoassay tests
are more practical than NP swabs. In some cases, individuals
can self-collect their own samples. The disadvantage of
antigen testing is that it is less sensitive than PCR, meaning
that more virus must be present in the sample before it can
be detected. Patients who are asymptomatic may have lower
amount of virus present and antigen testing might produce a
false negative result.

The most widely used test is detection of viral RNA
using polymerase chain reaction or "PCR."   This is a
laboratory technique that was invented in 1983 by Kary
Mullis, a co-recipient of the Nobel Prize for the invention.
Dr. Mullis died in 2019, just a few months before the
outbreak of COVID-19, coincidentally of pneumonia. His

invention is used millions of time every day around the world for testing to help save lives. PCR is a nucleic acid amplification technique that is widely used as a tool for molecular research and diagnostics.

In humans, the genetic material is encoded into DNA. Various forms of human RNA functions as an intermediary in the cell's function to produce proteins. Like many other viruses, the genetic material of SARS-CoV-2 is encoded

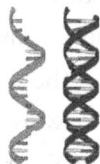

RNA DNA

within its RNA sequence. Unlike DNA which consists of two complimentary strands, RNA is single stranded. DNA contains four bases named adenine, guanine, cytosine, and thymine. For RNA, uracil is substituted for the thymine base. Humans are more complex than viruses and bacteria and require much more genetic material. Our DNA are incorporated into pairs of chromosomes. The proteins we produce come from the blueprints of our parents. The coronavirus contains only one strand of RNA, and there is no inheritance.

Detection using PCR requires conversion of the RNA into a DNA clone prior to multiplication to get more copies. Probes that are labeled with fluorescent-colored dyes are used to detect the presence of specific regions of the coronavirus' molecular sequence. Amplification is conducted through in an instrument known as a "thermocycler." Each cycle consists of heating the DNA to accelerate the production of DNA copies followed by a cooling down period. These are known as cycles. This heating and cooling process is repeated. The number of cycles required to obtain a positive result is recorded. A sample devoid of the virus will fail to produce a signal after 40 cycles, and the test is terminated. PCR tests can take several hours to produce a result.

There are newer molecular tests that use faster and less expensive amplification methods, such as loop-mediated isothermal amplification or LAMP. This is an alternate method of amplification of nucleic acid is that is much faster than PCR, and is useful when fast results are needed, e.g., a severely symptomatic patient who presents to the emergency room. The LAMP technique is conducted at a constant temperature (typically 60-65 °C eliminating the time needed to cycle the reaction chamber temperature (i.e., heating and cooling). Unfortunately, these tests are not as sensitive as PCR (Kashir et al.). Therefore, as with many things in medical science, there are trade-offs. Here, an individual who has a low level of coronavirus may produce a false negative test result. This is not an ideal situation as this individual may unknowingly infect others. A misdiagnosis may also lead to the initiation of the wrong treatment or delay in the initiation of the proper medical care.

Recently, the FDA has approved home collection and at-home testing devices. Distribution of these tests will allow us to determine our up-to-the minute virus status. This could be helpful if we want to travel for business, or to meet family or friends. The accuracy of at-home testing is likely to be less that what is achieved by certified laboratories (Axell-Houst, et al.).

Samples can also be tested for the presence of the viral proteins or antigens that are shed into the human body. These viral proteins are measured using immunoassays. This technique was invented in 1959 by Doctors Berson and Yallow, who also won the Nobel Prize for their discovery. Immunoassays use antibodies to specifically bind to their target. These antibodies are produced as part of an animal's immune defense response after the inoculation of foreign proteins, and thereby used as a reagent in immunoassays. After an infection, SARS-CoV-2 proteins are released and measured by this method.

All individuals who test positive are reported to the local or state Department of Health. A widely used indicator of a geographic region's growth or control of a virus is the "Rt" value. This is defined as the average number of people who become infected from exposure of a single infected individual. A Rt value greater than 1.0 indicates that the virus is spreading, while a value less than 1.0 indicates that the virus is being contained. During the pandemic, daily Rt values are reported by governmental health agencies. Early in the pandemic, it was not uncommon to see Rt values between 1.5 to 2.0, indicating a surge. The terms, "flattening the curve" is used by local, state, and national officials to indicate their desire to reduce the infection rate, which can be accomplished by sheltering and distancing of the population, e.g., closing gyms, beauty salons, proving education remotely instead of in person, and restricting dining to outdoors only. When the Rt value drops below 1.0 for a given region, it is used as signal by health officials that these restrictions can be reduced, e.g., opening schools for in person instruction and allowing indoor dining, and opening other non-essential businesses that are associated with have high interpersonal contact. The rate of test positivity among all tests that are performed is another indicator of current infection control. This figure was falsely high during the early months of the pandemic, as testing was restricted to symptomatic individuals due to shortages in testing supplies.

Testing for COVD-19 antibodies

Most individuals infected with coronavirus will develop "antibodies" that circulate in blood within a week or 10 days after an infection. Antibodies are produced by mammalian species from B-cells found in the bone marrow. The process begins with exposure to a microorganism that the body's does not recognize. The coronavirus is not a natural part of our makeup therefore our immune system labels its viral proteins as "foreign." A Martian visiting the earth is foreign and our first inclination is to defend against it. Antibodies are the defense weapon against foreign invaders. They are proteins that are shaped like the letter "Y." The bottom of

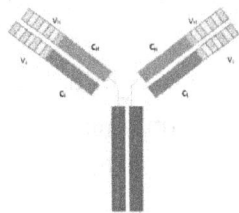

the antibody is known as the "Fc" portion and is produced by all antibodies. The two top wings of the letter Y are known as the Fab portion. This is the part that binds specifically to the foreign protein known as an "antigen." Like other proteins, antibodies are encoded with the host's DNA. The specifications of most proteins are specified by the DNA's sequence. Antibodies are different in that the different parts of its structure are produced separately and later assembled to make the final product.

There are several types of antibodies that differ in structure, location, and function, and are produced at different times. The IgE antibody is produced when an individual is exposed to common allergens such as pollen or peanuts. The IgA antibody is found in mucous membranes such as the nose. The majority of the antibody are found in blood and are of the IgG type. In general, IgM antibodies develop earlier after an infection than IgG antibodies although for a COVID-19 infection, the difference in antibody appearance is only a few days. There are also non-neutralizing and neutralizing coronavirus antibodies. The non-neutralizing antibodies include those directed against the virus' envelope. These proteins do not participate in the replication of the virus and are therefore bystanders. Neutralizing antibodies bind to the spike protein and block entry of the virus to the host cell. These antibodies have more clinical value than non-neutralizing antibodies when managing an individual who has been infected with COVID-19.

An individual immune status, i.e., protection against a future infection, cannot be determined by detecting the presence of COVID-19 antibodies in blood alone. It is true that the higher the antibody concentration, termed "titers", the more likely they are immune. The best test to determine if a person's antibodies are protective against a future infection is use of the "virus neutralization assay." In this test, cells are grown in a Petri dish that are treated with antibodies from a patient's serum sample. Then the cells are transfected with active coronavirus. If the antibodies are able to block entry of the virus into the cells, they are termed neutralizing. This test requires several days to perform. Due to its complexity, the virus neutralization assay is not routinely available within hospital laboratories. Moreover, working with live virus is hazardous and testing must be conducted in the appropriate biosafety precautions. Biosafety level II are lab procedures that are design to protect workers who handle specimens such as swabs or oral fluid that contain the virus. For the virus neutralization test, there is a higher exposure to live virus and requires biosafety level III procedures.

Antibody testing is not as important as virus testing from an infection control standpoint. It can be used to diagnose an infection from an individual who does not exhibit symptoms. Unlike other viral infections such as hepatitis, coronavirus antibodies decline a few months after an infection. The precise duration of COVID-19 antibody duration in blood is not yet known because the pandemic is new.

Other testing modalities for COVID-19 infections

In addition to antibodies, human immunity also consists of a cellular response. "T-cells" originate from the bone marrow and thymus and are cytotoxic, meaning that they can destroy invading cells. Coronavirus will stimulate mobilization of T cells to fight off an infection. Like antibody production, T-cells require 7-10 days to mobilize after viral exposure. Some of these cells also have memory, in that they stay longer after an infection and are available to guard against a reinfection. The role and value of T-cell function for use in the COVID-19 pandemic has lagged behind PCR, antigen and antibody testing. T-cells are measured using a specialized laboratory instrument known as a flow cytometer. These tests are being developed for use in clinical practice, but are currently used only for research purposes.

Within a hospital, there are specific findings on the chest CT scan that is characteristic of the pneumonia produced by the virus. While the American College of Radiology does not recommend CT scans for diagnostic purposes, they can be helpful when the PCR test negative and there are other clinical signs of a COVID-19 infection. Interpretation of CT scans require highly trained radiologists.

Economics for COVID-19 testing

The economics of testing is essential to understand

why there has been a shortage of testing supplies. This has been an important factor in the escalation of the COVID-19 pandemic. Many have asked, "If we don't know who is infected, how can we know who to quarantine?" Many have also wondered why it has taken so long to develop tests. As described in the previous paragraph, testing for SARS-CoV-2 is difficult. It is not like taking a drop of blood from a fingerstick and putting in onto a strip to get a reading in seconds, as is the case for glucose.

Due to the shortage of supplies, reference labs that have a high volume of COVID-19 testing considered using "sample pooling" (CDC). This refers to mixing multiple samples together and testing them as one. The CDC has provided guidance to this procedure. If the mixture tests negative, then all samples contributing to the pool are reported negative and no further work is needed. If the pool is positive, the individual samples used to compose the mixture are individually tested to determine which one (or more) triggered the positive result. Sample pooling can save use of precious reagents. As an example, if 100 samples are tested, pooling 5 samples together would require 20 analyses. If the positivity rate is 10%, there will be 2 pools that would reflex to individual testing, requiring reagents for 10 more samples. The net result is a savings of 70 tests per 100 samples received. The disadvantage of pooling is that each sample is diluted reducing the sensitivity of the test by a factor equal to the number of samples that are combined. For mildly positive and possibly asymptomatic individuals, a false negative result might result that can have significance to spreading the pandemic. There are also more expenses for the labor involved. Therefore, pooling has not been adopted on a large scale.

Shortages of COVID-19 tests are directly related to the investment the U.S. has made into diagnostics. Prior to the COVID-19 pandemic, the worldwide gross income for the in vitro diagnostics industry, responsible for clinical laboratory is estimated at $60 billion, with the US market purchasing about 40% of that figure. This covers billions of lab test on several thousand different analytes (In contrast, the income for the pharmaceutical industry is 25 times that amount).

As described in my story chapter, "Lab Heroes," the Affordable Health Care Act further resulted in the passage of PAMA, that further reduce our country's investment in clinical laboratory testing. The reimbursement for clinical laboratory tests by Medicare and Medicaid were reduced by 20% in 2018. These cuts were necessary to provide money to insure individuals under the Affordable Health Care Act who did not have insurance. This reduced the ability of the In Vitro Diagnostics (IVD) industry to produce new clinical laboratory tests needed to combat COVID-19, and to clinical labs to implement these tests.

To understand what it would take to test everyone, consider these figures. The typical cost for COVID-19 virus testing is approximately $100. If the entire US population of 330 million alone were to be tested just once, the $33 billion cost for testing would exceed the annual US expenditures for the entire IVD industry. In April 2020, the Administration approved $25 billion specifically earmarked for COVID-19 testing. When this was used up, an additional $75 billion was requested in November 2020 for more testing and contact tracing. This stimulus package will provide access to testing and the long waits to get results will be a thing of the past. Recently, the FDA has approved an at-home COVID-19 test. This promises to be a major step forward in providing access to testing needed in curtailing the pandemic.

Even with this financial support, there is and continues to be fierce competition for testing supplies between laboratories and even between States of the Union. We have witnessed test kits being "bartered" to the highest bidder. As a provider of healthcare for sick patients, it is my biased belief that the priority should be given to hospitals, medical centers and clinics. What we have seen, however, is that some industries, e.g., airline travel, can spend more money for COVID-19 testing, and therefore manufactures of testing kits have diverted product to these away from our clinical needs. In a time of global pandemic, inconvenience for non-essential functions should not be at the expense of increased morbidity and mortality. We have also seen other examples of inappropriate profiting. Early in the pandemic, price gouging has occurred for essential personal protective equipment. For example, the price for N95 respirators from some vendors increased over 1000%.

On a smaller scale, price inflation has also occurred with the clinical lab. There are brokers who obtain clinical samples of COVID-19 positive blood that are sold to manufacturers for their use in developing assays. During the early stages of the pandemic, it was not uncommon to see that these brokers sold samples at significantly inflated prices. While this may not have been illegal, it certainly was unethical.

In March of 2020, President Trump issued an Executive Order 13190, entitled, "Preventing Hoarding of Health and Medical Resources To Respond to the Spread of COVID-19." Among the items listed as "scarce" and therefore subject to this order included masks, respirators, face shields, gloves, gowns, and other personal protective equipment, ventilators, disinfectants, sterilizers and sterilization services. Despite this Order, these practices will occur again when there is a new crisis.

References

Axell-Houst DB, et al. The estimation of diagnostic accuracy of tests for COVID-19: A scoping review. J Infect 2020;81:681-97.

Centers for Disease Control and Prevention. Interim guidance for use of pooling procedures in SARS-CoV-2 diagnostic, screening, and surveillance testing. https://www.cdc.gov/coronavirus/2019-ncov/lab/pooling-procedures.html

Kashir J, et al. Loop mediated isothermal

amplification (LAMP) assays as a rapid diagnostic for COVID-19.   Med   Hypotheses   2020; doi: 10.1016/j.mehy.2020.109786

COVID-19: Medical Issues and Treatments

****

Home remedies and prophylaxis

The popular media is replete with reports of home drugs and vitamins that can be taken to reduce the likelihood of a COVID-19 infection. Most of these suggestions and recommendations are not supported by randomized clinical trials. The absence of scientific data does not disprove the value of these medications. Conducting preventative clinical trials is very expensive, because large numbers of subjects must be enrolled to demonstrate a benefit. Moreover, pharmaceutical companies have no incentive to pay for a trial for a generic drug. These clinical trials would have to be funded by government grants. Therefore, the evidence presented that suggests efficacy is based on retrospective observational data from infected individuals. There can be biases in the interpretation of the data, and the level of evidence is lower than from a randomized clinical trial.

As an example, vitamin C is one treatment that may be useful in protecting an individual from a COVID infection. Also known as ascorbic acid, vitamin C is an antioxidant. Vitamin C is water soluble, inexpensive, widely available over the counter, and has no side effects. Prior to the COVID-19 pandemic, clinical trials have shown that those who have low levels were more susceptible to respiratory infections. Retrospective analyses of COVID-19 infected patients have shown that ascorbic acid levels are lower in non-survivors versus those who lived (Zhang et al.). There are prospective studies underway to determine if vitamin C can be used to treat infected patients. Until results of randomized trials are reported, the value of taking vitamin C to prevent a COVID-19 infection is unknown.

Similar comments can be made regarding the value of other available over-the counter treatments aids commonly used to fight the common cold. Zinc is an essential heavy metal for cell division, growth, and healing. In a retrospective study in Spain, 249 patients with COVID-19 were studied (Vogel-Gonzalez et al.). Patients with a zinc level below 50 µg/dL had worse clinical outcomes, with prolonged length of hospitalization (25 versus 8 days). These investigators also showed that SARS-CoV-2 replicates better in cell cultures deplete with zinc.

The importance of maintaining a minimum concentration of vitamin D for overall medical benefits has been touted for decades. It is not only essential for bone health, as vitamin D also has anti-inflammatory properties. One of the biggest proponents is television star and talk show host Oprah Winfrey, who revealed in 2009 that she had a vitamin D deficiency. As stimulated by her broadcast, we in the clinical laboratory received a surge of requests for measuring the vitamin D levels in blood that has continued to this day.

Individuals who have vitamin D levels below 30 ng/mL in serum are said to be "deficient," while people with less than 20 ng/mL are "insufficient." Vitamin D exists in two forms, D2 and D3. They are equally useful biologically. Vitamin D comes through diet (milk, cheese, etc.), and sunlight exposure. The skin absorbs ultraviolet B rays from the sun which converts 7-dehydrocholesterol to vitamin D3. For people living in the northern latitudes where the sun angle is less direct, low vitamin D levels are common, especially in the cloudy winter months of the year, when individuals tend to stay indoors. Even during the summer, many individuals use sun block to reduce risk for developing skin cancer, and in doing so, block the conversion of vitamin D production. Individuals who have dark skin pigmentation produce less vitamin D from the sun as melanin inhibits its production.

The correlation of vitamin D levels and severity of COVID-19 infections has been studied (Jain et al.). Among the 154 COVID-19 patients studied, those with a vitamin D deficiency had a 21% mortality rate versus just 3% for those with normal levels. There was an inverse correlation between serum vitamin D concentrations and biomarkers of inflammation, such as ferritin, interleukin-6, and tissue necrosis factor-alpha. As with the other supplements, there are no randomized clinical trials that demonstrate its effectiveness against COVID-19. Unlike vitamin C, chronic excessive intake of zinc can cause anemia and a reduced immunity, while too much vitamin D can produce bone and kidney problems.

Another substance that has been studied for COVID-19 is melatonin, a hormone found in the brain. It has been used as an aid to world travelers who have to adjust to different time zones. With regards to COVID-19, treatment with melatonin may be beneficial to critically ill patients who are treated with ventilation. Melatonin reduces blood vessel permeability inducing sedation, decreasing agitation and increases sleep quality. A study conducted at the Cleveland Clinic showed that individuals who used melatonin had a 28% lower likelihood for a positive PCR test for COVID (Zhou Y, et al.). Even more dramatic was the finding that among African Americans, the likelihood was reduced by 52%. This is one of the few studies that showed a medication could reduce the risk of an infection. Taking melatonin, however, could affect sleep cycles from the non-traveler. And these days, who is really traveling let alone overseas? Loss of sleep is harmful for individuals who are infected with viruses or bacteria.

Treatment of infected patients

There have been many different therapies attempted to treat critically-ill and non-critically ill patients suffering from COVID-19. One of the more publicized treatment failures was hydroxychloroquine. This is a drug used to treat arthritis and malaria. It was hoped that the drug's anti-inflammatory effects would be effective on COVID-19, given that these individuals have significant amount of inflammation (Global Virus Network).

Some severely ill COVID-19 patients suffer from a phenomenon known as the "cytokine storm." This is when a person's own immune response goes overboard and instead of being protective against an infection, it potentiates it. "Tocilizumab" is a monoclonal antibody that blocks the receptor for interleukin-6 activity (IL-6). The use of tocilizumab was studied in a randomized trial of 161 patients compared with 81 placebo controls (Stone et al.) There was no difference in the outcomes in preventing intubation or death and the trial was terminated.

Convalescent plasma was also extensively studied. This treatment involves collecting plasma of individuals who have a COVID-19 infection. It was hoped that these antibodies produced by a donor after in an infection and present in convalescent plasma could block entry and propagation of the coronavirus when the plasma is given to an infected recipient. Convalescent plasma therapy was first used to treat patients infected with influenza during the 1918-1920 Spanish flu outbreak. It has been considered for flu treatment today but has not been adopted (Luke et al.). Unfortunately, in a randomized clinical trial of 228 COVID-19 patients who received the plasma, there was no difference in the rate of adverse events and mortality when compared to those who received a placebo for critically ill patients (Simonovich et al.). This has been confirmed by other studies as well. It may be used early in a COVID-19 infection.

Antiviral agents are widely used for treating patients suffering from other viral infections such as human immunodeficiency virus (HIV) and hepatitis C. Remdesivir is an inhibitor of RNA polymerase, a key enzyme needed in the replication of coronavirus. This antiviral agent has been successfully used in treating SARS-CoV-1 and the Middle East respiratory syndrome, at least in the laboratory. In the Adaptive COVID-19 Treatment Trial, 521 patients received the drug in a double-blind trial (Beigel et al.). (A "double-blind" study means that neither the subject nor the investigator knows if the patient is receiving the target drug or a placebo, i.e., an inactive pill that looks the same.) Hospitalized individuals infected with SARSoCoV-2 and evidence of a lower respiratory tract infection, remdesivir improved clinical outcomes, shortened the time to recovery, reduced serious adverse events, and reduced overall mortality.

In other trials, the combination of remdesivir along with dexamethasone has shown promise. This combination has been recommended for treatment of COVID-19 patients by the National Institute of Health (NIH). Dexamethasone is a synthetic steroid that has been used for many years for the treatment of arthritis and allergic skin reactions. This combination is widely used although there are currently no randomized clinical trials demonstrating efficacy.

Treatment with monoclonal antibodies raised against the coronavirus have become another means to treat

COVID-19 infections. Also known as "biologics", these antibodies are produced through recombinant DNA technology where a gene is inserted into a different organism's genome, so that it can produce that particular protein according to its sequence. Monoclonal antibodies produced in this manner are designed to bind to the spike protein of the virus. This blocks the binding to the angiotensin converting enzyme-2 (ACE2) cell surface receptor, and thus the virus cannot gain entry into cells containing this particular receptor. While this doesn't block the virus' entry within an individual, it prohibits the its proliferation.

In general, antibodies that are used for treatment or diseases have long, complicated, and difficult to pronounce names. Pharmaceutical companies have adopted a convention whereby the suffix, "-mab" identifies the drug as being antibody based. For the generic name of the drug, these companies use names that are difficult to pronounce or remember. This is done purposely so that their trade names are used instead. For example, trastuzumab is a biologic drug used to treat patients with breast cancer. The tradename, Herceptin, is much easier to remember, especially since the first part of the name, "her" refers to females, and the latter part, "ceptin" refers to binding to the Her2 receptor. When a drug company's patent expires giving rise to less-expensive generic versions, the drug's chemical name is retained. The pharmaceutical company who produced the original drug hope that doctors and patients will continue to ask for the original drug through its tradename. There is a convention that scientific reports should use the drug's chemical name.

For patients with mild or moderate COVID-19 infection, the FDA has approved casirivimab and imdevimab, which are to be used in combination with each other, and bamlanivimab to be used alone (Eli Lilly). These treatments are not designed to be used for severe or hospitalized patients. There will likely be other monoclonal antibody-based treatments to come.

Once an individual is infected with COVID-19, treatment is gauged on the severity of the disease and availability of hospital resources. At various times during the pandemic, there have been shortages of intensive care unit beds, personal protective equipment like gloves, gowns, and masks, qualified doctors and nurses, ventilators, and nasopharyngeal swabs. The discussion in this chapter is largely informational, and not meant for patients and their family members to have a large role in treatment decisions. As a non-physician myself, I would never advise anyone as to the proper choice of therapy. COVID-19 is a new disease with treatment strategies changing month by month. Physicians and infectious disease specialists are on the front line of this disease and they are in the best position to make critically important life-or-death medical management decisions. It is not prudent to over-ride their experience and qualification.

When President Trump tested positive for a

COVID-19 infection in early October 2020, shortly after his first debate with the Democratic candidate, Joe Biden, he was treated with a combination of remdesivir, dexamethasone, a two-monoclonal antibody cocktail (Regeneron), and melatonin, while admitted at the Walter Reed Medical Center in Washington DC. It is unclear how much of the treatment decisions were influenced by the President himself. One hopes that he did not use his own infection and decisions regarding his care to set an example for his own policies for political gain. It is remarkable and perhaps lucky for his age and weight that his infection took a mild course and he quickly survived to return to the campaign trail.

Artificial breathing

Many individuals who are infected with COVID-19 become severely ill and have extreme difficulties in breathing. In order to survive, these patients may first be given 100% oxygen (normal room air contains 20% oxygen). If that is insufficient, they may be treated with mechanical ventilation or intubation. This is a process where a tube is inserted into the trachea or windpipe. In order to paralyze the diaphragm, the individual is placed under an anesthetic such as the drug propofol. Oxygen can be funneled through the breathing tube and into the body, and a separate tube is used to remove harmful carbon dioxide. An individual may be intubated for many days or longer.

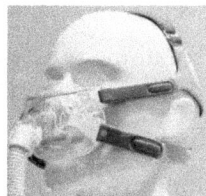

An alternate manner to assist in breathing is the use of extracorporeal membrane oxygen or ECMO. This device takes blood out of a patient, adds oxygen to the blood and returns it back to the patient. It is considered as a "last ditch" treatment for patients with respiratory problems. ECMO requires highly skilled and trained individuals and is not available in all medical centers. The success rate of intubation and ECMO is roughly 60%. There have been shortages of ventilators as well as ICU beds and staff during various stages of the pandemic.

Clinical laboratory tests indicative of poor outcomes

SARS-CoV-2 affects many systems of the human body. This dysfunction can be detected by conducting routine clinical laboratory tests. Patients who have difficulty breathing are tested for arterial blood gases. Severely ill patients will exhibit low oxygen content, a high carbon dioxide level and an alkaline pH. Those who have cardiac injury will have increased concentrations of troponin, a protein that released from the heart. There are also increases in d-dimer, a test that indicates the excess presence of blood clots. Inflammation is a key consequence of a SARS-CoV-2 infection. This causes the release of inflammatory markers such as C-reactive protein (CRP), interleukin-6, and ferritin Zhou F, et al.).

Long term health effects

It has been estimated that 10% of infected and

symptomatic individuals who survive a SARS-CoV-2 infection will suffer continuing medical issues lasting for months. Some who contracted the SARS CoV infection (the earlier version of coronavirus) in 2003 had continuing medical issues years later. These chronically diseased and impaired individuals are termed, "long haulers." As one would expect, older individuals and those with pre-COVID-19 morbidities are most likely to suffer from chronic effects. These problems cause both direct damage by the virus, and indirect damage as a consequence of the infection. Structural damage to the heart, as assessed by cardiac imaging, can lead to heart failure and an irregular heartbeat (known as cardiac arrhythmia). Patients with a SARS-CoV-2 infection have an increased tendency to form blood clots, the cause of myocardial infarction, pulmonary embolism, and cerebral vascular accident. Lung disease due to the permanent loss of alveoli may experience persistent breathing problems, with smokers being particularly at risk due pre-existing lung damage and inherent decrease in oxygen delivery to the body.

There can also be a decline in cerebral function, with memory loss and mood changes such as depression. The cost to the healthcare system of managing these patients adds to the burden of treating acutely infected patients. Financial support from governmental agencies will likely be required for the millions of COVID-19 disease survivors with chronic problems. This is a topic that has not been considered or discussed.

References

Beigel JH, et al. Remdesivir for the treatment of COVID-19. Final Report. N Engl J Med 2020;383:1813-26.

Global Virus Network. Progress in the treatment of COVID-19. https://gvn.org/progress-in-the-treatments-of-covid-19/

Jain A, et al. Analysis of vitamin D level among asymptomatic and critically ill COVID-19 patients and its correlation with inflammatory marker. Sci Reports 2020; doi.org/10.1038/s41598-020-77093-z

Lilly's neutralizing antibody bamlanivimab (LY-CoV555) receives FDA emergency use authorization for the treatment of recently diagnosed COVID-19. Available at: https://investor.lilly.com/news-releases/news-release-details/lillys-neutralizing-antibody-bamlanivimab-ly-cov555-receives-fda.

Luke TC et al. Meta-analysis: convalescent blood products for Spanish influenza pneumonia: a future H5N1 treatment? Ann Intern Med 2006;145:599-609.

National Institute of Health. Therapeutic Management of Patients with COVID-19. https://www.covid19treatmentguidelines.nih.gov/therapeutic-management/

Zhang J, et al. High-dose vitamin C infusion for the treatment of critically ill COVID-19. Pulmonology 2020; DOI: 10.21203/rs.3.rs-52778/v1Peng

Simonovich VA, et al. A randomized trial of

convalescent plasma in Covid-19 severe pneumonia. N Engl J Med 2020; doi: 10.1056/NEJMoa2031304

Stone JH, et al. Efficacy of Tocilizumab in Patients Hospitalized with Covid-19. N Engl J Med 2020;.org.DOI: 10.1056/NEJMoa2028836

Vogel-Gonzalez M, et al. Low zinc levels at clinical admission associates with poor outcomes in COVID-19. medRxiv doi.org/10.1101/220.10.07.20208645

Zhou Y, et al. A network medicine approach to investigation and population-based validation of disease manifestations and drug repurposing for COVID-19. PLoS Biology 2020; https://doi.org/10.1371/journal.pbio.3000970

Zhou F, et al. Clinical course and risk factors for mortality of adult inpatients with COVID-19 in Wuhan, China: a retrospective cohort study. Lancet 2020;395:1054-62.

Immunity and Vaccines

****

Contact tracing of previously infected subjects

An important method to curb any pandemic is 'contact tracing.' According to guidelines established by the CDC, when an individual tests positive for an infectious microorganism like SARS-COV-2, test results must be transmitted to state, tribal, local, or territorial health authorities within 24 hours. These include tests for the virus, viral antigens or antibodies. Public health scientists, in turn, have the responsibility to find all the individuals who have been in contact with that infected person, to determine the origin of that infection. Timing is essential to the success of contact tracing to curb infections, especially for infected individuals who are asymptomatic (Kretzschmar et al.). If tests are not conducted quickly or results reported timely, the infected individual can unknowingly infect others after that first contact. Once an infected person is identified, health officials can enforce a quarantine of that person, usually for 14 days. Other individuals who came into contact with the infected individual can be called in to be tested and quarantined if necessary.

During the first month of the COVID-19 pandemic in the U.S., several individuals who were on luxury cruise ships became infected. Even before lab testing was available to confirm an infection, it was necessary to isolate those symptomatic individuals and trace their contacts. This was an ideal situation because when these passengers were at sea, they could not disperse beyond the ship itself. Once docked, COVID-19 testing was conducted before any individuals who were negative for the virus could be released from the ship.

There are some individuals who believe that contact tracing violates their rights of privacy as American citizens. They have stated that individual rights does not supersede public safety. Many objected to the Nation's shelter-in-place mandates that occurred in the spring of 2020, and they refuse to wear masks in public today. As an individual working in the key part of the healthcare system, i.e., lab testing, I am opposed to the attitudes these individuals have. While I respect the right for everyone to have and express their beliefs, I also subscribe to the notion that during the times of crisis, sacrifices must be made for the common good. We have seen other generations that have faced and accepted personal sacrifices, such as rationing of products that were required of civilians during World War II.

Herd immunity

Limiting the spread of the COVID-19 pandemic begins with "herd immunity." This is defined by a large fraction of a community being immune to a virus. The creation of a vaccine is the best approach towards achieving herd immunity. Normally it takes many years and even decades to create and globally distribute a vaccine. Even if the existence of the bacteria or virus is well known and characterized, the development of a vaccine is not guaranteed. To date, there is no vaccine to human immunodeficiency virus despite a worldwide effort to create it, and no vaccine for tuberculosis, which was first described in 1720.

Herd immunity can also be achieved by purposely inducing infections to a population and producing a natural immune response. In order to halt the pandemic, it has been estimated that 70% of a population would have to be exposed and rendered immune. While this strategy has been suggested as a strategy for curbing COVID-19, it is not a realistic option. In attempt to maintain its economy, Sweden attempted to produce herd immunity among its citizens early in the pandemic by minimizing the restrictions on its citizens. This approach was initially successful, it eventually caught up to them. In December 2020, this country had a much higher rate of confirmed cases and deaths compared to its neighboring Nordic countries.

Many individual's infected with SARS-CoV-2 will perish from an infection. Some proponents would argue that only the elderly would die, it is clear today that individuals of all ages are at risk for a COVID-19 death. Even those who survive, there is no guarantee that the individual will be free from a re-infection, or from infection by a new strain. So even in societies that cherish the young, this is not an acceptable strategy.

Vaccine history

With the high morbidity and mortality of SARS-CoV-2, there has been an international effort to create a vaccine and to accelerate its use. Unfortunately, concerns for vaccine safety has been raised for the initial COVID-19 vaccines. It is unfortunate that vaccine development became a political issue during the presidential campaign. The Trump Administration wanted to take credit for the progress of the vaccine leading many U.S. citizens to believe that safety measures were compromised in the rush to show progress in vaccine development prior to the election. Given that the FDA has regulatory processes that cannot be countermanded by the White House, safety issues were not sidelined. Unfortunately, even under normal circumstances, adherence to the influenza vaccine administration among adults was less than 50% during the 2018-2019 season. Therefore, we cannot expect that the majority of the population will be immune, until perhaps years after release of the vaccine.

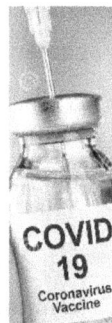

Edward Jenner, an English physician, who in 1798, was the first to create a smallpox vaccine for cows. He is credited for saving countless lives. According to the World Health Organization (WHO), only two viruses have every been completely eliminated from the earth: variola that causes smallpox and the non-human rinderpost virus, which infect cattle, domestic buffalo, giraffes, and other large mammals. The last major polio pandemic in the U.S. occurred in 1952 where there were over 57,000 cases and more than 3000 deaths. With the development of the polio vaccine, the number of cases dramatically declined with no new cases originating from the U.S. since 1979. While two of the three polio strains have been declared eradicated, there are a few new cases each year coming from Afghanistan, Nigeria, and Pakistan. Currently, the WHO has licensed 25 vaccines that are used worldwide.

Vaccines are biological materials that are injected into the host to illicit a natural immune response. The vaccine itself is usually an agent that either resembles a disease-carrying microorganism, is a weakened form of the microbe, or one that has been inactivated. The immune response that protects the host from an infection is in the combination of antibodies and T-cells. Antibodies against invading infectious against can be continuously produced for years and even decades. For example, researchers in the 21st Century have found antibodies in circulation from individuals who have been exposed and survived the 1918 influenza outbreak. Cellular immunity also can persist for long periods of time with the production of "memory" T-cells.

The COVID-19 Vaccine

There are many pharmaceutical companies who have developed vaccines against SARS-CoV-2 and they are in various phases of clinical trials and approval by the FDA under their Emergency Use Authorization. Two companies, Pfizer/BioNTech and Moderna have developed vaccines against SARS-CoV-2 using a unique approach that has not been tried before. Their vaccines contain a modified version of messenger RNA, with a sequence that encodes the coronavirus's receptor binding domain (RBD). The vaccine injected into a subject's skeletal muscle. The modified mRNA is encapsulated into a lipid nanoparticle which enables it to cross the lipid membrane of the human cell and into the cytoplasm. Once there, the host muscle cell begins to produce the SARS-CoV-2 RBD protein according to the mRNA sequence. After this viral protein is made, it is released into the blood where it stimulates an antibody response, similar to what occurs during a natural SARS-CoV-2 infection. There is no chance that an intact virus can be produced from the vaccine, as the injected mRNA sequence is for only one of the many viral proteins that comprise an intact and living virus, and is not alive by itself.

The mRNA method for vaccine development was first conceived in the 1990s by Katalin Karikó, a Hungarian-born scientist who was at the University of Pennsylvania. While her theory that specific mRNA sequences can be used by a host to produce foreign proteins, there was a stumbling block that prevented it from working in humans. The mRNA would be recognized by the host and destroyed before it could work. With the collaboration of Drew Weissman, also at UPenn, the pair produced a modification of the mRNA that took longer for the cell to recognize it before it was inactivated. The promise of new drugs based on mRNA lead to the formation of two companies, Moderna based in Cambridge, Massachusetts, and BioNTech, based in Mainz, Germany, and where Katalin Karikó joined as a senior vice president. When the pandemic hit, both companies switched their operation towards producing a COVID-19 vaccine. Their mRNA method accelerated the timelines as never seen before in the history of human vaccinations. If the mRNA COVID-19 vaccines are successful in producing herd immunity, many believe that Drs. Karikó and Weissman will eventually be awarded a Nobel Prize for their scientific discovery. They will follow other notable scientists whose theories were rejected and funding for their research was difficult to achieve.

Pfizer/BioNTech (Sahin et al) and Moderna (Jackson et al.). received FDA EUA clearance for their vaccine in December 2020. The effectiveness of these vaccines against COVID-19 were determined in Phase III trial to be 95%. In the BioNTech trial of 43,000 participants, there were only 8 subjects who were given the vaccine developed COVID-19 as compared to 162 from the placebo arm (95.3% effective). There were no fatalities and only 3.8% complained of fatigue and 2% complained of a headache. This vaccine is directed to the receptor binding domain (RBD), part of SARS-CoV-2 spikes, and was demonstrated to produce both positive antibody and T-cell responses. The average amount of IgG antibodies produced were higher than the amount found in individuals who recovered from a COVID-19 infection. One issue with this vaccine is the requirement that it be stored at -70°C.

Similar results were obtained from the Modera vaccine. In their 30,000-participant phase III trial, there were 5 individuals who developed COVID-19 out of the 95 total (94.7% effective). One advantage of this vaccine, however, is that it does not require -70°C storage. This effective rate was higher than predicted. As with many vaccines, the one for COVID-19 requires a booster injection a few weeks later. There may be some individuals who do not return for a second injection if they experienced side effects from the initial inoculation. These individuals may not be adequately protected by the vaccine against a COVID-19 infection. At this date, it is too early to determine the duration of the antibody immunity.

As a healthcare worker, I was offered and received the Pfizer/BioNTech COVID-19 vaccine within a few weeks of its availability. I was one of the fortunate ones that did not feel any side effect during either the initial or booster injection. I am lucky in that I have never had a bad reaction to any of the vaccines I have taken during my youth or as a professional.

During the Pfizer and Moderna vaccine trials, there were two deaths among those who took the vaccine and four who received the placebo. Outside of these trials, there have been other individuals who have died shortly after taking a COVID-19 vaccine or the booster shot. The retired baseball slugger Henry Aaron died on January 22, 2021, 17 days after accepting a COVID-19 vaccine. Some of these individuals had comorbidities and may have passed due to natural causes and their deaths were coincidental to the vaccine itself. There was no medical evidence that Aaron's death was linked to his vaccination. There have been a few reports of younger, apparently healthy individuals who have passed. This has led some people to refuse accepting the vaccine. The overall death rate, however, is extremely low and the vaccine by most medical experts is considered very safe.

On February 27, 2021, Janssen Pharmaceuticals (better known as Johnson & Johnson vaccine, the parent company) received FDA clearance for their viral vector vaccine. This company used the more traditional viral vector method that is in common with other vaccines such as for influenza. Instead of using mRNA, in this approach, a small segment of the adenovirus is replaced with the SARS-CoV-2 gene for the spike protein. When administered, the host produces the protein which in turn, stimulates the immune system to produce antibodies. In clinical trials, the FDA found this vaccine to be 72% effective in preventing a COVID-19 infection, slightly lower than the Moderna and Pfizer vaccines. It was reported to be 82% effective at preventing severe disease. The advantage of this vaccine is that it does not need cold storage and only one dose is required.

SARS-CoV-2 strains

Infectious diseases such as influenza, are able to survive on the planet because of their ability to change or mutate. These minor changes to the nucleic acid sequences occur through the process of natural selection. A mutated virus that can escape eradication by treatment or blockage by human antibodies will survive at the expense of the virus that is not adaptable. This is "survival of the fittest," a phrase coined by Herbert Spencer after he read Charles Darwin's theories on evolution in 1864. Various forms of coronaviruses have been in existence infecting humans and animals for over 100 years. Over time, these viruses survive by adapting to their environment. The original severe acute respiratory (SARS) virus came on the scene in 2003 and infected 8000 individuals in China. The Middle East respiratory syndrome coronavirus (MERS) infected 2500 individuals.

Specifically, regarding SARS-CoV-2, a critically important question to all of us moving forward is, "Does a prior infection to SARS-CoV-2 make me immune to a future infection?" Because we don't know how long antibodies and T-cells remain in circulation, the answer to this is unknown. At the current time, the re-infection rate is extremely low. Re-infection is defined as somebody who initially tests positive, recovers, develops antibodies, and consistently tests negative for the presence of the virus, and then turns positive for the virus at some future time, e.g., months or even years. There have been isolated case reports of individuals who test positive after a prolonged period of time (months) of negative results (Tillett et al.). Genetic studies have shown that these individuals have a slightly different genetic strain, i.e., the virus has mutated. Perhaps the antibodies raised against the initial infection are still present but are no longer effective. It may also be that the antibody titers have declined over time to render them less effective. In either case, a high re-infection rate will enable this virus to survive beyond the current pandemic.

What is known about the current SARS-CoV-2? From the short time of its existence, this virus has undergone one major viral mutation. It has evolved to be much more infectious and difficult to contain than its predecessors. As the world knows, it originated in Wuhan, China and came to the U.S. where the first cases were seen in Washington State. The genetic sequence of this virus was quickly performed, and the virus was labeled by some virologists as the "Washington Strain (Korber et al.)" As there were many airplane flights from China to the West Coast of the US, this was the predominate version of the coronavirus infection during the early months of the pandemic. About the same time the virus was infecting Washington and California, a mutated version of SARS-CoV-2 was making its way to Italy and Iran. This virus had mutated to a different form and was labeled by the virologists as the "European Strain." It wasn't long before flights from Europe arrived on the East Coast of the US infecting metropolitan areas, especially New York City. Within a few weeks, the country was put into a lock down mode, with international flights canceled and imposed severe domestic travel restrictions. Infections continued to mount over the coming weeks and months. By May, 2020, when it appeared that the rate of infections started to decline, the country was in a deep recession with high rates of unemployment. As the country slowly opened its doors for travel and business, there was a second serge of infection.

In November 2020, two and possibly three new strains have been identified. Each of these appear to be more transmissible than the previous version. The "B117" mutation was first detected in the United Kingdom and has spread to other countries in Europe, Middle East, Asia, and Australia. A second strain has been labeled "501Y.V2" and originated from South Africa and is believed that it too may be more infectious than the others before it. Mutations are part of the virus' mission for survival. It is hoped that the virulence of new coronavirus mutations will be less lethal. Since the objective of any organism is survival, the death of its host is not a favorable outcome for the virus either. There are other factors that affect the death rate, such as healthcare resources. Therefore, it is too early to determine if these mutations are less lethal.

Small changes in the viral genome is termed "antigenic drift." These changes modify the viral proteins that are encoded by the nucleic acid sequences. Mutations can modify the ability of the host's immune response, such as with antibodies or T-cells. "Antigenic shift" refers to major changes of a viral genome and their resulting proteins, creating new subtypes. For example, one subtype may infect primarily one animal species, e.g., bats, and mutates to the extent where it can now infect humans.

The influenza virus is a good example of both antigenic drift and shift. Over the centuries of its existence, this virus has undergone many minor mutations or drifts. The occurrence of an antigenic shift can result in the creation of pandemics. There have been many influenza outbreaks despite the existence and use of vaccines.

The creation of a SARS-CoV-2 vaccine may cause or accelerate further mutations of the coronavirus. If the European strain is curtailed with widespread vaccination, the virus may mutate to a new strain. If the U.S. is among the first to adopt the vaccine on a wide population-based scale, the new strain might originate here. In that case, it might be called the "American strain." Labeling of strains according to the geographic location has been used for political gain and is inappropriate. Some politicians have labeled SARS-CoV-2 as the "China virus." This contributed to the polarization of the nation. Perhaps if a new coronavirus is detected, it should be labeled SARS-CoV-3?

References

Korber B, et al. Spike mutation pipeline reveals the emergence of a more transmissible form of SARS-CoV-2. doi: https://doi.org/10.1101/2020.04.29.069054

Kretzschmar ME, et al. Time is of the essence: impact of delays on effectiveness of contact tracing for COVID-19, a modelling study. MedRxiv 2020; https://doi.org/10.1101/2020.05.09.20096289

Jackson LA, et al. An mRNA vaccine against SARS-CoV-2 – Preliminary Report. N Engl J Med 2020; 383:1920-31.

Sahin U, et al. COVID-19 vaccine BNT162b1 elicits human antibody and Th1T cell responses. Nature 2020;586:594-9.

Tillett RL, et al. Genomic evidence for reinfection with SARS-CoV-2: a case study. Lancet Infect Dis 2020; doi.org/10.1016/S1473-3099(20)30764-7

The Apprentice

****

My secretary buzzed me on my phone.

"You have a call from the White House," she said.

"Do you have a miracle drug to fix my hair? It has got to be a prank," I said. "Did they give you a name?"

"The woman said it was somebody by the name of Dr. Foechy," she said. "Should I hang up?"

"One second," I told her. *Foechy, Foechy, who sounds familiar, but where do I know this name?* I thought. *Fauci!*

"I'll take the call!" I said to my secretary. She transferred the call and soon I was talking to the head of the National Institute of Health Institute of Allergy and Infectious Diseases.

"The President wants you come to DC right away. He wants to you to head a team of lab scientists to compete against another team for technologies for COVID-19 testing," Dr. Fauci said.

"Why me?" I asked.

"We know that you have expertise in validating immunoassay testing platforms. This new virus is affecting Wuhan, China, and the President wants to get a handle on it in case it comes here," he said.

"That's wise. We are all hoping that this will not be a big issue. The SARS COV-2 infection also started out in China in 2003, but it was quickly contained. My understanding is that there were only a handful of cases in the U.S.," I said.

"Twenty-nine in America, to be exact," The director said.

"But what do you mean by a competition?" I asked. SARS stood for Severe Acute Respiratory Syndrome-Associated Coronavirus. Since the original virus was identified in 2003, this new strain was listed as "2." SARS-CoV-2 is responsible for the disease, COVID-19.

*

After cancelling all of my appointments, I arrived at Reagan National Airport the next day. Except for my wife, I didn't tell anyone where I was going. At baggage claim, there was a man carrying a sign with my name on it. There was no indication that he was with the White House. I checked into the hotel near 1600 Pennsylvania Ave. The next day, I was taken to the West Sitting Hall on the second floor. There was a woman seated there.

"My name is a Daniela Bass. I am the director of the Microbiology Lab at Johns Hopkins University."

I introduced myself as a clinical lab director and sat down next to her. "Do you know what this is about?" I asked.

"Something about a competition." Dr. Bass was interrupted. We both stood up immediately. Into the room came President Donald Trump, Mr. Henry James from the

State Department, and Dr. Anthony Fauci. Trump is taller and thinner than I imagined. I guess they are right about what television does to people's images. The doors to the Sitting Hall were closed. The three of them remained standing, as did we. The President was in the middle, Mr. James to his left and Dr. Fauci to his right. They were all dressed in business attire.

"Welcome to the White House. This is an amazing place. Henry is from my Cabinet. This is Dr. Anthony Fauci of the NIH. Antony is a terrific scientist. He thinks that the corona virus will be a pandemic and I want to get ahead of the curve. So, I am setting up a competition. Each of you will head a team. Dr. Bass, your team will focus on novel technologies to detect an active infection."

Turning to me, he said, "Your team will set up an antibody assay to determine immunity. Pick a name for your team, and select your staff. You will each have a $1 million budget. You will present your ideas and prototype assays to us in two weeks. The winner will be the first 'Technology Apprentice.' Dr. Fauci will give you the details. Now go."

Before we left to return home, we were asked to pick names for our team. Daniela's group was known as "Team Detect." My team was called, "Team Immune."

*

Unlike The Apprentice television show, it was not possible to develop a lab test at a suite in the Trump Tower. I flew home and immediately began thinking about how I was going to develop this test, and what novel technology I might create to impress the judges and the POTUS in order to win the competition. When I got home, I immediately assembled my team of local experts. There wasn't time to recruit people to come from other parts of the country. Within a day, Team Immune consisted of Craig Varmus, the chief microbiologist from our clinical lab, Tzeng Liu, a protein chemist from our University, Robert Zupperman, an assay development scientist from a laboratory diagnostics company in the city and Candice Berger, marketing person from a local advertisement agency. I knew and trusted all of these people on my team from prior work that I had done. I assembled the group in our conference room and had our initial strategy meeting.

"The President has asked us to create a lab test that can be used to determine immune status of subjects infected with the coronavirus. Is that possible in the next two weeks?"

"I will defer to Robert, but won't it take months to raise the antibodies needed for this test?" Candice asked.

"Normally, yes, but if we can get some of the viral protein itself, this will be sufficient to immobilize antibodies in the blood," Robert said. "Tseng, how difficult will it be to purify the antigen?" Everybody knew that the antigen is what attracts antibodies from a blood sample.

"That could take weeks to months in itself. Fortunately, my former mentor is in Wuhan. I spoke to him today and he is sending us the spike protein to SARS-CoV-2 for us to use, as we speak," Tzeng said. "Normally it is difficult to import such products, but I can get the State

Department to grant us special privileges for this project," I told the group. "I have also arranged to have serum samples from people confirmed to be positive for COVID-19 that we will need in order to test for the presence of antibodies."

"As controls, we can obtain serum from our influenza patients," Craig remarked. "Plenty of those samples in my lab now."

"We still need to develop something that will make the judges realize how important this is. A test that has to be done in a lab and takes hours will not win. Candice, what did you have in mind?"

Candice unveiled a plan that was challenging technically, but appealing for a potential mass audience. I told every one of my intended timelines and milestones and dismissed the group. "There will be daily morning meetings to discuss the progress and resolve bottlenecks."

Then Candice asked, "If we lose, will we have to go to the oval office and be fired by Mr. Trump?"

"Never mind that. Get to work," I said as I was getting up and leaving.

*

In Baltimore, Dr. Bass and Team Detect created a similar team of scientists from academia and the in vitro molecular diagnostics industries. In many ways, her task was more technically difficult, because testing for virus counts requires more analytical steps. A test for COVID-19 requires extraction of RNA from a patient's sample. Initial studies from Wuhan showed that a swab to either the throat or nasopharyngeal cavity are the specimen of choice and not blood. The isolated nucleic acid needs to be multiplied, and then the measurement of the viral content can take place. I knew it would be difficult for her to find specimens from infected patients, as there were very few patients with this virus in the U.S. at the time. She might not have the connections overseas that we had. The need for fast diagnosis was also more important for her test than ours, which is designed to determine immunity after an infection. She would have to invent new testing methodologies which can take months or years. I felt pretty good about our chances to win. Dr. Bass and her team quickly formulated a plan. In order to enact this strategy, they added a noted mechanical engineer to the team. This was not somebody we didn't have or even think that we needed.

*

The work went on at a feverish pitch. All of my research studies were put on hold in favor of this one project. I took a sabbatical from all clinical, administrative, and teaching responsibilities. My group stayed late each night and came back to work early the next morning, and worked through the weekend. Nobody complained, and everybody was excited by the prospects of producing something meaningful for the nation's well-being. We all hoped it wouldn't be needed. Little did we know that very soon, our work would be put to the real test. We knew that on the other coast, our corresponding counterparts were working equally hard. Nobody outside my department knew about this competition. When the work was done, we were all exhausted but pleased at what we accomplished. I hoped it would be good enough.

*

Within two weeks to the day of my initial visit to the White House, I was back with my senior team ready to disclose our results to the President and his judges. That morning, I arranged to have a cordial breakfast with Daniela Bass in the hotel. Like me, she looked very tired and worn, but excited at the same time. We did not talk about projects. I learned that she was a mother of teenage children and I asked her about them. She said she had not seen much of them over the past two weeks, but her husband and kids were supportive of her efforts. I said the same about my family.

Team Detect and Team Immunity arrived at the White House and were put into the West Sitting Hall. The presentations will be made in the East Sitting Room. Team Detect was chosen to go first. I felt in some ways, this was an advantage for them, because they could explain to the judges what COVID-19 was and why it could be a national emergency. Neither team would be able to listen to the other team's presentation. Afterwards, we would be stating our case for why our team should win.

Dr. Bass entered the East Sitting Room with her team. There was a camera man and a studio director present in the room. The usual furniture was set aside and a large corporate-type desk was in the middle of the room. There were five chairs on one side and three chairs on the other.

Dr. Bass and four of her colleagues stood by their seats on one side. Within a few minutes, Henry James and Anthony Fauci arrived and stood to the left and right of the middle chair. Then a door behind the room opened, and President Donald Trump entered. He was smartly dressed with a customed-embroidered shirt and sporting a solid red tie. He sat down in the middle seat and motioned everyone else to be seated. He then asked Team Detect to begin.

Dr. Bass started. "COVID-19 is a virus that can produce flu-like symptoms to infected individuals. We are hopeful that this virus will not spread to the U.S., because we don't really have effective therapies and there is currently no vaccine yet to make people immune. If it does come, we think that containment will be important to protect our citizens. This requires rapid identification of COVID-infected individuals, and quarantine of positive cases for two weeks. Effective medical management will require access to viral tests that are accurate and fast. Our current tests for other viruses can take 3 hours to produce. Our concept is three-fold. First, we miniaturized the testing device so that it fits in a physician office instead of a lab. Second, we reduce the time required for testing to just 5 minutes for positives and negatives. And third, we plan on establishing stations throughout the city where people can drive up and have their nose swabbed while they are in the car, and give test results before they leave. To further minimize risk of infections of our employees, we have created Max. A robot who can do the sampling without exposing the collector." A diagram of

Max was shown to the judges. "Max cleans itself with bleach after every patient. After collection, Max turns and drops the swab into the test device and within 1 hour we have results. We need to take COVID seriously and develop contingency plans for worst case scenarios. In Wuhan, they have prohibited travel, locked down the city, and restricted gatherings for all of its citizens. I hope that doesn't happen here."

Then the President spoke. "That's fantastic Dr. Bass. Your team has done an amazing job. Let's now hear from Team Immunity."

It seemed Team Detect was in there for an hour, but in reality, it was only 15 minutes. We got the summons to appear, my heart started racing and my breathing got labored. I was a little unsteady when I arose, but I quickly recovered and led my team to the East Sitting Room, passing Team Detect in the hallway. My eyes caught Dr. Bass'. She looked relieved and confident.

Knowing that it would be redundant to Team Detect's description of the current COVID-19 situation, I focused on the need for antibody testing. "If we face a pandemic in our country, virus testing will definitely be important to make the correct diagnosis and isolate positive patients from infecting others. The next step in this chain of medical practice will be to determine who has been exposed and who is immune from future exposure. There are two antibodies that we are testing. The IgM produces first, usually within a few days after infection. This is followed by the conversion to IgG production a few days later. Eventually, the IgM antibody goes away and we are left with the IgG antibody. By testing both antibodies, we can determine approximately when the individual was infected and when they may be immune. There are some prototype assays developed in China. They have not been evaluated as to their neutralization ability."

"What does that mean and why is that important?" President Trump asked.

"Antibodies can be directed against any viral protein but that does not mean a person is immune. Our assay is directed against the spike protein that blocks the virus' entry into our cells. This will be able to determine if an individual is immune from a future infection. This test will also be useful to monitor the success of vaccines. The experience from Wuhan is that most people infected with COVID-19 will not experience symptoms and will not know they were infected. They may unknowingly infect people who they come in contact with. Wuhan has taken the stance that we can't test everybody so let's just quarantine the entire population. What makes more sense for America, is to test people for the presence of the antibody using an inexpensive, fast, and readily available blood test. We hope that asymptomatic individuals who have antibodies using our test will be immune and can return to their jobs."

"Show me what you have." The President asked.

"We have developed a finger-held testing device for COVID antibodies. It is like a urine pregnancy test. One drop of blood and within minutes you have an answer. You don't have to wait an hour to get results. It is inexpensive and can be done by anybody with just a minimum amount of training."

After a round of questions from President Trump and his advisors, he thanked and dismissed my team. He asked for Dr. Bass to enter. The two of us took turns fielding questions from Dr. Fauci.

"How long will it take to get regulatory approval? How long will it take to produce these products? Can this model of testing be used in the future for other infections yet to come?"

Then the President asked, "If I had enough money to fund one, why should we pick yours?"

Dr. Bass answered. "I believe you need to start with anyone who has an active infection and then go from there. We have to test all individuals who have symptoms."

"Pretty compelling argument," the President said. He then turned to me. "What can you offer?"

"Mr. President, we will need both technologies to keep our citizens safe," I said. I think the robot is an unnecessary expense. We can do this work with our medical staff, given the proper personal protective equipment. I have taken the liberty of contracting a company who helped us develop this test. They have produced enough strips to test 100,000 today. Here is a video of the production line that I took yesterday. We have arranged with the Chinese government to have these kits sent to Wuhan right now. If and when we need them here, we can produce large quantities within a day or two. All I need from you, sir, is emergency provision from FDA to release these products.

The President asked Dr. Bass and me to step outside while he discussed the two proposals with his judges. When we returned, he gave the verdict.

"I've never done this before in my television shows, but this is real life. The nation owes you a debt of gratitude. You have both won. We need both lab tests so congratulations. Go back and start production of your kits for Americans. But Dr. Bass, hold off on the robot for now." She nodded her head. I shook the hands of everyone in the room, had our picture taken, and left the White House. *I hope we don't need this,* was my parting thought.

*

The COVID-19 virus is closely related to a coronavirus found in bats. The initial cases of COVID-19 appeared in December 2019 in Wuhan, China. Many of the first individuals to become infected visited the Huanan Seafood Wholesale Market, who sold live animals for consumption. From there, the rate of infections doubled each week. During the Chinese New Year, infected Wuhan citizens traveled to other cities infecting others. The Chinese government locked down the entire country resulting in containment of the virus. Unfortunately, infected individuals traveled to other parts of the world causing widespread infections throughout.

In America, early infections occurred in Seattle and Santa Clara County of Northern California. To minimize infections, this led Trump to lock down the entire population. International travel and large gatherings of people were prohibited. The initial lab tests for COVID-19 were developed by the US Centers for Disease Control and Prevention. But they were unable to supply clinical laboratories with a sufficient amount of test kits to meet the needs of the escalating rate of infections. Unlike this study, the current antibody tests have not been evaluated against immunity status. Therefore, a next generation antibody test is needed.

Prior to becoming President of the United States, Donald Trump was the key figure in the television show, The Apprentice and Celebrity Apprentice. Contestants were divided up into two groups and given tasks to promote a product or raise money for charity. Each team presented their project to Trump, who decided a winning group and fired one individual from the losing team. When there were only two contestants left, the show had a final task where one individual was crowned the winner. The show was very popular with many seasons and spin off shows. After Trump's election, former California Governor Arnold Schwarzenegger was the host replacing Trump. There was no competition between teams for COVID-19 test development. The inability to obtain test kits facilitated the spread of COVID-19 to unsuspecting citizens worldwide. Now that President Trump has lost the election, will there be new episodes of The Apprentice?

Shelter-in-Place

****

Sylvia worked in the front office of a construction company right out of high school. She landed the job with help from her grandfather, Charlie, who worked for this company for many years as a foreman. The company specialized in erecting new office buildings and laboratories for biotechnology startups. Franco, one of the electricians at the firm, took a liking to Sylvia and they started dating. He was playful with Sylvia telling her corny jokes and funny stories. She liked him because he wasn't always so serious like the others were in the office. Sylvia looked forward to seeing him come into the office every day. A few months later, Sylvia moved in with Franco and later that year, she became pregnant. Sylvia was part of a large family with three brothers and four sisters. Most of them lived nearby so there were always many nieces and nephews around during family gatherings. Sylvia was thrilled to be starting her own family with Franco.

Sylvia continued to work in the office during her pregnancy. Midway through her second trimester, the COVID-19 pandemic struck the nation. She along with other non-essential businesses were ordered to close and the employees were instructed to shelter-in-place at home. Sylvia didn't mind this, as she was experiencing some difficulties with her pregnancy. Franco was also not allowed to come into work for fear of the virus spreading so he was at home as well. The two of them became ever closer, having to spend all of their time together.

"It's terrible that I can't see my family right now," Sylvia remarked to Franco. "But we have to be especially careful. We wouldn't want anything to happen to our unborn child," she said. At the time, the effects of the coronavirus virus on fetal health was largely unknown, and naturally, they did not want to take any chances.

Dr. Harriet McCormack was Sylvia's obstetrician. During these times, she arranged pre-partum visits with Sylvia through video internet connections, rather than exposing Sylvia to her other patients. Dr. McCormack stressed the importance of hand washing and minimizing exposure to other people. Sylvia complied and essentially never left the house. When Franco left the home to buy groceries, he wore an industrial mask that he used when working construction.

Sylvia and Franco's plan for a large wedding were postponed due to the pandemic. Rather than waiting, the couple learned that the state granted virtual weddings. The marriage license application was completed, and submitted online. The only requirement was they both attend and have at least one witness present.

Regarding these requirements, Sylvia made a

comment to Franco. "Really? It is not obvious that both of us need to attend? Is there something more important that your future wife or husband has to do? Honestly!"

"Hey, I was thinking about marrying our next door neighbor without asking." Franco said. "She's really hot."

"You go ahead and do that if you want," Sylvia said.

Then Franco grabbed an empty beer bottle, turned it upside down, held it to his mouth, and started singing an old Beatles song. "I want you. I want you so baaaaaad. I want youuuuu. I want you so baaaaaad it's driving me maaaaad, it's is driving me mad."

"Cute," Sylvia's said. "Find out where we can buy toilet paper. We're almost out."

He started singing again. "If I must longer I must linger, I will have to use my..."

"Get out!" was Sylvia last response.

Once the paperwork was processed, and a date was scheduled, the two married. Family members participated via web conferencing.

In early May 2020, the county determined that construction work was deemed essential and Franco was permitted to return to work. After a few days on the job, Franco came home one day with a cough and muscle discomfort. His job wiring circuits sometimes requires him to fit into very tight spaces in between walls. While he is used to minor aches and pain, these symptoms were a little different. He called in sick the next day when his symptoms worsened. He was now suffering from a low- grade fever.

Sylvia wanted him to go to an urgent care medical facility but Franco was hesitant.

"How do you know I won't catch COVID-19 while I am there?" he asked his wife.

"It might be too late. I think you already have it," Sylvia said. When his symptoms worsened the next day, he left the house and went to the General's emergency department. He told Sylvia to stay home and not accompany him.

*

Our emergency room has an isolated triage area where patients are separated from each other. The room is disinfected after each patient visit. Everyone wears N95 ventilators and personal protective equipment. Mounted on the wall is a hand sanitizer dispenser that was used between examinations of each patient. Next to the sanitizer was a curious device that had a 2- inch circular cavity. Franco wasn't sure what that was until one of the doctors briefly put the head of his stethoscope into the device. When the scope was removed, the device had automatically applied a protective barrier onto the diaphragm piece. Franco recognized this was a procedure that prevented the stethoscope from contaminating the next patient to be examined. His notion was confirmed when he saw the product label, "Aseptiscope." Franco felt his fears lessened as it appeared that catching COVID-19 was really low at this hospital.

After an initial examination, Dr. Harvey Rosenberg,

the ED doctor assigned to Franco, said that he needed to be tested for a COVID-19 infection. He told Franco what to expect and then opened a nasopharyngeal sampling kit. Dr. Rosenberg inserted the long nasal swab deep into Franco's nose. It was very painful to Franco, causing his eyes to tear up. Our laboratory offers a variety of methodologies to meet the testing needs for the virus. Some of our assays require 3 to 5 hours for completion but can simultaneously measure nearly 100 samples at a time. Other assays can produce results within 5 to 45 minutes, but each sample must be tested one at a time. In Franco's case, the doctor ordered the testing stat. The result would determine if he was infected by the coronavirus or if additional workups would be necessary to explain his symptoms. Within an hour, our laboratory reported that Franco was positive for the virus responsible for a COVID-19 infection. Dr. Rosenberg decided to discharge Franco because his symptoms were not serious enough to warrant admission. It was also a move to protect other patients and his staff from an unnecessary infection risk.

"I am ordering a 14-day quarantine from your work. I see that you are married. Is there anyone else living with you and your wife?" Dr. Rosenberg asked.

"No, just her. She is 7-months pregnant. Is there any danger to the baby she is carrying?" Franco asked.

"Because you came after the onset of symptoms, she and her fetus may already be infected. Please have her come in as soon as possible and we will test her," Dr. Rosenberg said. "Then we can make a plan of action."

Franco called Sylvia immediately, and went home to pick her up and return to the ER. Two hours later, she arrived and Dr. Rosenberg ordered a COVID-19 test on her. Although she was not symptomatic, she too tested positive, and the couple were discharged to self-quarantine.

While sheltered, Franco and Sylvia watched the national news each night hoping to gain insights on how patients with COVID-19 can be treated. In particular, Franco was concerned about whether the virus might cause birth defects. He found a blog written about it by the State of New York Governor's sister-in-law.

"Sylvia, check this out. Cristina Cuomo, who has COVID, is taking bleach baths in hopes of neutralizing the virus. I think we should try this," Franco said to his wife. "It should kill any virus we have in our bodies."

"Are you nuts? Bleach is very dangerous. I am not going to do that!" Sylvia was adamant.

But Franco was undeterred. The next morning, he went into the laundry room and put one half cup of Clorox into their bathtub full of water and soaked in it. Sylvia awoke to the smell of bleach and immediately went into the bathroom.

"Franco, get out of there now! You may be hurting yourself," she said. "I told you not to do that. Honestly! I wonder about you sometimes."

"Hey, even the President said that when disinfectants get in the lungs, it knocks out the virus in just one minute," Franco said.

"The chlorine won't stop there. It will knock out your lungs too." Sylvia reached into the water and pulled the drain plug. She then got a towel and her husband reluctantly got up and out of the tub. "Don't do that again."

"Yes, dear," Franco muttered somewhat sarcastically. Franco was lucky and did not suffer any ill effects from this medically unproven idea.

*

With that episode aside, the remainder of Sylvia's pregnancy was unremarkable. When her contractions started to be more frequent, Franco brought her to our Labor and Delivery area. Sylvia's obstetrician ordered a repeat COVID-19 test. The sample was sent to my lab and we performed the testing like so many others we receive each day, but this one was different. Most COVID-19 virus tests look for two separate portions of the gene for the virus' nucleocapsid protein, labeled N1 and N2. Both must be present for the test to be positive. When only one is positive, the result is considered "indeterminate." This is what occurred in Sylvia's most recent sample. As per our protocol, the original specimen was retrieved and re-tested using an alternate methodology. The repeat test produced the same result. When Dr. Rosenberg received the result, he decided to re-test Sylvia by swabbing her nose again. This time, the result came back positive. The next day, Sylvia delivered a healthy baby boy with good Apgar scores. Sylvia remained in the maternity ward for two days before she and their newborn were discharged. Dr. Rosenberg told the couple that the repeat COVID-19 positive test result was due to the presence of remnant viral particles that were episodically released from her tissues and that she was not actively infected. The baby tested negative for the virus.

"You can breastfeed your child," Dr. Rosenberg said to Sylvia. "Get lots of skin contact, especially early on." He did state that other family members should stay away from the family if any of them had any symptoms suggestive of a COVID-19 infection.

*

While providing laboratory services is the main part of my job, learning more about diseases and how new tests can be used for better diagnoses in the future is an especially rewarding part of my profession. During this pandemic, my research laboratory helps companies develop new COVID-19 assays. One project is to evaluate an antibody test to determine if a previously exposed individual is immune against a future infection. I scheduled a meeting with my research group and the study sponsor to summarize some of our initial findings.

"Thanks to your efforts and those of others, we now know a lot about how COVID-19 antibodies develop in infected patients. As seen with other viral infections, patients with COVID-19 will produce three different types of antibodies. The IgA and IgM antibodies appear with 7-10 days after an infection. The IgG antibody comes along a few days after that. We have seen similar appearance patterns for other viruses like hepatitis B. After a few months, the IgM antibody begins to decline and IgG remains for years if not decades. But unlike hepatitis, we have seen that the IgG also begins to decline after just a few months. This is not good news, because we don't know if the presence of antibodies necessarily indicates that an individual is immune from future infections."

"Whoa! How does that happen?" Carla, one of my techs asked. "I thought the purpose of antibody production is to ward off infections. Now you are telling me that there is no guarantee of that?"

I responded. "Antibodies are produced against foreign proteins. The coronavirus has several of these. Some of these proteins are structural in that they hold the virus together. Since none of these viral proteins are normally present in our bodies, they are recognized as foreign, and we produce different antibodies against each protein. The spike protein, however, is the key as this is how the virus binds to our tissue to propagate the infection."

"They call it a coronavirus because the spikes on the surface resembles a crown," Carla remarked.

I never understood the analogy. *The virus is spherical and has thorns throughout. A crown is not a ball but a glorified hat with protrusions.* Then somebody else in my lab spoke up.

"No Carla, it is called corona because it resembles a solar corona," he said.

"Irrespective to origin of the name, the important thing is spikes. An antibody that can bind to this protein might be able to block the virus' entry to our cells," I told the group. "The presence of the other antibodies indicate that we have been exposed but they do not necessarily protect us, so, it depends on how the antibody blood test is constructed. For an assessment of immunity, it is essential that you choose the right target protein for testing."

"The receptor binding domain of the spike protein!" Carla asked.

I was impressed that Carla had done her homework on this topic. "Correct," I said. "Due to the pandemic nature of coronavirus, the FDA created an "emergency use authorization" for tests involving corona virus and antibodies. There is no requirement that they demonstrate immunity. Perhaps that will be important for future assays," I said.

"How do we prove that serum antibodies are in fact neutralizing?" she asked.

"You compare results from COVID-19 positive patients against a test called the "virus neutralization assay." The test involves incubating antibodies from that patient with cells grown in a Petrie dish. Then by adding live coronavirus we can see if the antibodies can prevent spread of the virus. This test takes days to perform, so it is not practical to use routine clinical labs today. It is also extremely dangerous test, as working with live viruses can infect lab workers."

"I've seen news stories showing techs working in these labs. They look like astronauts. Carla said. She saw a vision of herself in one of these protective suits, with the face shield all fogged up and having breathing problems. When she came to, her body shuddered at the thought.

I then brought up a particularly disturbing issue to my group and Dr. Fred Wingate, a research scientist employed by the manufacturer of the lab test. "In reviewing clinical data, we came across a pregnant woman who tested positive for the virus using our lab's PCR test during her 8th month. She didn't have symptoms and was instructed to shelter at home. A week later, her repeat test was negative. When she delivered her child one month later, her PCR test was unexpectedly turned positive. The antibody tests were not available from 5 weeks ago, and today, we only have the results from your prototype assay."

"What did you find?" Dr. Wingate asked.

"A very puzzling antibody profile. Her IgM is marginally positive and her IgG was negative," I replied.

"If the patient was positive for the virus while pregnant, and she is still positive today, why aren't the antibody levels higher now? She had plenty of time to mount a response from her first infection," Dr. Wingate asked.

"I see three explanations for these findings. Some patients who are immune suppressed or are taking an immunosuppressive drug and therefore are not able to produce any antibodies. Maybe she is one such person," I remarked.

"But the test revealed IgM, the antibody that usually comes out first, is mildly positive. Could it be that her original antibodies cleared and this is an indication of a new infection?" Dr. Wingate asked

"Yes, that is a second possibility," I responded. Then I hesitated before proceeding.

"And the third reason," Dr. Wingate wanted to know.

"Your test produced an error," I said. Dr. Wingate didn't like that answer but he acknowledged that this was possible.

"Shouldn't we alert her physician of the possibility that her current virus positive result could be signs of a re-infection? Or at least ask him to order the test officially so it can be reported and acted upon?" Dr. Wingate inquired.

"Morally that might be correct, but because your test is not FDA approved, the medical research board will not permit a report of an un-validated and possibly erroneous result to either the patient or their provider. Ethically, they cannot even know that we used the patient's specimen for research purposes." I said, begrudgingly.

"There is potential for harm in reporting an incorrect test result as well, not to mention the legal quagmire this establishes." But we were both thinking the same thing. *What if the result was right? She could be infecting others.* This dilemma kept me up at night for many days after our discovery. If I reported these results, my research could be shut down, my reputation stained, and my livelihood jeopardized. In the end, I felt I could not intervene.

*

The experimental antibody test were from Syvia's blood. Sylvia tried to control who were allowed to visit her, Franco and their new baby. When visitors and well-wishers came, they were all asked not to hold the baby and to wear a mask at all times. When her grandfather Charlie visited, his personal protection practices were less than optimal. He didn't wash his hands as frequently as he should have and his mask would occasionally fall below his nose. Four days after his visit, Sylvia's grandfather, Charlie, became symptomatic for COVID-19. Due to his advanced age and the fact that he had diabetes and hypertension, he died three weeks later. It was unclear how he contracted COVID-19. Sylvia and Franco were not able to say goodbye to Charlie in person. The funeral was held via a teleconference. Our research group could not determine if Sylvia was the cause of her grandfather's infection.

*

Human research is supervised by Institutional Review Boards, or IRBs to prevent unauthorized experiments, like those that were conducted during World War II by unwilling subjects. Testing of samples sent to clinical laboratories for routine testing can be conducted without authorization by the patient or physician, as they are deemed to have no biological risks to the subjects themselves. Because test results can be wrong, the data cannot be released to caregivers, who make inappropriate medical decisions. When biological samples are collected for the sole purpose of the research and are not leftover from clinical testing purposes, consent is required by the subject. However, the subject is notified that the same restrictions apply with regards to release of unproven data.

As of this writing, it is unclear how often an individual who has recovered from his or her initial coronavirus infection can become re-infected. Remnant viral particles can resurface after a period of dormancy. Molecular testing for the virus is the gold standard for the initial diagnosis of a COVID-19 infection. Unfortunately, it is currently not a good test for detecting a re-infection. An assessment of virus viability requires growing the virus in a culture. Individuals handling live viruses are at risk for an infection, and such work is carefully conducted in level three biosafety hoods. Thus, it is not a widely available procedure.

The value of serum antibody testing remains somewhat elusive. At best, results can determine if an individual has been exposed to coronavirus. However, incorrect interpretation of results can have significant societal consequences. A positive antibody test result might lead an individual to relax their guard thinking that they are immune when they are not. Until it can be proven that an antibody test confers immunity, it is still best to exercise caution. This is particularly true when interacting with individuals who are at high risk for developing COVID-19 medical complications following an infection. A negative antibody test result likely means no infection within the prior 7-10 days. But it may be possible that an infection occurred months ago and that the antibody titers have declined.

Worldwide, the rate of documented re-infections have been low, to suggest that the antibodies that we are producing are protective. Alternately, the pandemic hasn't been around long enough for immunity to wane in a given person. Recent research has suggested that there are at least two SARS-CoV-2 strains in America. While all of the novel coronavirus originated from Wuhan China, the one that migrated to the State of Washington was the most common form found in the early months of the pandemic from infected patients living on the West Coast. Conversely, a mutated form known as the "European strain" appeared in Italy and Iran, and became the predominant form found on the East Coast. Today, the European SARS-CoV-2 strain is the only form that can be found in the Continental U.S. Time will tell if antibodies to the Washington strain will prevent an infection by the European strain. As of this writing, there are additional mutations that have surfaced in the United Kingdom and South Africa and may be more contagious that its predecessors. Probably by the time you read this, they will have arrived in America.

Lab Heroes

Rada was the only child of Thai family who immigrated to the United States to Northern California when she was 5 years old. Rada, which means "with care," was a good student and wanted to become either a doctor or a nurse. Unfortunately, her family did not have enough money to send her to college. After high school, she enrolled into phlebotomy program, and received her license after completing a 40-hour course, and performing 50 supervised sticks through an externship program in my laboratory. She received her California license. Rada stood out among the other students, and we hired her immediately after she qualified for her license. Her work ethic was superior and over the years, she became our most reliable blood collection technician. When we had a patient who was difficult to collect blood from, we would call Rada. When we needed blood from small children, intravenous drug addicts who had poor veins, and the elderly who had thin and frail skin, we called Rada. When we needed blood from the psychiatric ward, we called Rada. Sometimes these patients would become belligerent, but Rada had a very calm demeanor and would take the time to explain the procedure, and why obtaining their blood was so important. This helped put patient's mind at ease. There were times when she was verbally abused, and one time was nearly physically assaulted, but it did not deter her from doing her job each and every day. When you find people with this work ethic, you hold onto them like it was the last person on Earth.

*

Prior to the COVID pandemic, I attended a fund raising dinner at my University for healthcare heroes. Among the awardees was a surgeon who performed an emergency procedure on a little girl who had fallen from a tree. The child and parents were at the reception honoring this doctor. The surgery was particularly difficult and took seven continuous hours. This was a particularly noteworthy procedure, as the surgeon together with a biomedical engineer from the University of California, Berkeley, had recently invented a new device that minimized tissue injury. He tried to explain it to the lay audience, but it went over their heads. Even I had trouble keeping up but was happy that this man was receiving recognition.

The doctor recalled that the team was totally exhausted after the surgery on that day.

"Everybody had sweat pouring out of their bodies, it was that intense. But when it was all over, and our patient made a full recovery, I took out my team for a celebration about a week later," the surgeon said to the audience.

In gratitude, the family gave a sizable contribution in honor of the team, which was used to expand the pediatric intensive care unit ward. In his acceptance speech, the surgeon thanked the other members of his team including the anesthesiologists, scrub nurses, other physicians and therapists who oversaw her recovery in the intensive care unit. He even thanked the cafeteria staff who provided meals that the child asked for before the procedure. Absent from these accolades was the role of the clinical laboratory, including the blood bank who not only provided packed red cells and fresh frozen plasma needed for the operation, and performed testing to ensure that the units that were safe. There were many other blood and electrolyte lab tests that was conducted by other members of my lab staff to monitor the progress of the surgery and the recovery of the child. While I was pleased that the doctor got the praise for his efforts, I was disappointed that he unintentionally excluded mentioning our team efforts. I didn't take any personal offense at this omission. After 30 plus years in the clinical lab field, I have come to expect that our efforts are largely taken for granted.

*

During the first weeks of the COVID-19 pandemic, there was a shortage of personal protective equipment. In particular, masks and face shields were in short supply across the country. Priority was given to doctors and nurses who were in the wards and had direct contact treating infected patients on a daily basis. Laboratory testing for COVID and non-COVID patients requires the collection of blood samples. Phlebotomists have limited exposure to a patient, as it generally takes 10 to 15 minutes to collected blood. In a given day, however, they may be dozens of patients. In many cases, the infection status of the patients that need blood collection is not yet known to the phlebotomist, at the time that a sample collection is needed. Phlebotomy is extremely dangerous occupation. The staff works with long sharp needles that can easily penetrate the skin. The inadvertent injection of a contagious pathogen can be fatal.

When the COVID-19 epidemic struck our hospital, Rada volunteered for extra duty. During the first few months, there was a shortage of N-95 masks, and phlebotomists were not offered this protection. They were given paper masks that were not as effective as the N-95. When the supply became adequate, about 6 weeks into the outbreak, Rada was one of the first in line to be fitted with an N-95 mask. She arrived at the appointed time for a mask fitting.

"Why is it called N-95?" she asked Sarina, a member of our infectious disease control staff.

"According to NIOSH, it filters at least 95% of all air particulates," Sarina said. Rada was instructed on how to don the mask properly. "Make sure you have the right side up," Sarina said. "The top strap goes on the back of your head just above your ears. The bottom strap is positioned around the neck below your ears. The straps should not cross. There is a metal clip on the top of the mask. Pinch this clip around the bridge of the nose to ensure a tight fit." Once the mask was in place, Sarina placed a hood over Rada's head.

"I am going to spry the inside of the hood with a sweet-smelling gas." After a minute, she asked if Rada could smell any of its aroma.

"No scent. I think I have it on right," was Rada's response. Sarina took the hood off, and taught Rada the proper means to remove the N95 mask.

"Never touch a used mask itself," Sarina said. "Discard it properly in a waste container. You should not use a mask for more than a few hours." Rada was now properly fitted and was ready to face COVID patients.

*

Rada knew that she was doing essential work for our hospital and that we really needed her. Sometimes I would see her at the end of the day, completely spent. She never complained, and she was always there at 6:00 am on the next morning. I had a concern that tired workers can make mistakes. In her line of work, this can be fatal. I had belief that Rada would know to stop or slow down if her mind and body began to wonder away from doing her job safely.

*

Beginning in early April, all of our healthcare workers were screened with forehead temperature checks and asked questions about our exposure to COVID patients and if we were suffering any symptoms. When cleared to enter the hospital, we received a sticker indicating that we had passed the screening process. If an individual had to leave the hospital during the day, for example to eat lunch, they can return without re-screening by showing the tag to the guard. Rada put her daily sticker on the back of her name badge. Soon, she had over a hundred stickers, layered one on top of the other. It became a badge of honor for her.

The laboratory analysis of samples from COVID-infected patients is also hazardous work. This is particularly true for testing nasopharyngeal swabs. These samples contain live virus that when inhaled, will produce a COVID-19 infection. Our laboratory staff are exposed to positive samples on a daily basis. There are precautions that are taken. The processing of swabs should be conducted inside an approved and certified biosafety cabinet. The testing of samples is often performed using large molecular diagnostics analyzers that cannot be easily operated within these hoods. The virus can be deactivated by heating or using a nucleic acid preservative known as DNA/RNA Shield.

*

As a clinical laboratory director, I get this question from reporters from time to time, "Why can't we provide the number of tests needed to satisfy the nation's demand for COVID?" A good part of the reason relates to the lack of respect that the clinical laboratory field gets from the public and legislatures. This was exemplified by the enactment of PAMA, part of the Affordable Healthcare Act. On January 1, 2018, the U.S. Centers for Medicare and Medicaid (CMS) published the revised clinical laboratory fee schedule, showing reductions in laboratory test reimbursements by 40-50%. For many of our laboratory tests, reimbursements are the life-line for the laboratory. Poor reimbursements meant that we have to reduce our expenditures, which usually mean staffing. This also has a trickle-down effect to the specific industries that support the clinical laboratory. PAMA meant that companies that make diagnostic equipment and reagents were experiencing less revenue from clinical labs. This resulted in an overall downsizing of the entire diagnostic healthcare industry.

I wrote an editorial to the local newspaper where I detailed the plight of the clinical laboratory with reference to decreasing reimbursements. I particularly highlighted a discrepancy between value and resources. "It has been estimated that 70% of all medical decisions are based on the result of a clinical laboratory test," I wrote. "Despite this metric, the clinical lab only receives 3-5% of the total operating budget." Usually companies invest in the areas where their product produce the most profit or value. It didn't make sense to me the clinical lab which is so essential to the success of a medical practice would get so little resources to it. I thought to myself, *would a shoe company ever spend most of their advertisement dollars on selling socks?*

I concluded the editorial by stating, "The COVID-19 pandemic has highlighted in an unprecedented manner the value of the clinical laboratory. The inability of getting accurate testing has led to the spread of viral infections by unsuspecting individuals. In retrospect, cuts to clinical laboratory reimbursements by CMS was not a good idea." The newspaper did not publish my opinion, or even acknowledge having received it. I sent to another daily paper across town but was ignored in the same manner.

*

I was hoping that this editorial would address the question of why we don't have enough tests. I usually respond as follows.

"The clinical laboratory industry has been cut to the bare bones due to reimbursement cuts. In the time of crisis, it takes time to bring back the scientific talent and manufacturing resources that companies were forced to discard or abandon. There was also a hesitancy to invest into producing hundreds of millions of test for fear, should the pandemic leave as quickly as it came. That hope was quickly dashed; we know now that the novel coronavirus will likely be with us for years to come," I said. They were largely unsatisfied by this answer. I think they were looking for somebody to blame. To this date, nobody in the media has linked the lack of testing capabilities to reimbursement cuts due to PAMA. But we on the front line of testing know that this was a major factor.

One month later, I was on my way to the hospital to start a new day when I noticed several police cars and fire engines in the front. There were also news trucks filming the proceedings. I gave it no thought until I got closer. One of the sheriffs, John Cannada, was somebody I had befriended years earlier. One of my research labs had been broken in by a psychotic emergency department patient who was high on methamphetamine. He damaged some of our equipment and threw files over the office. My research tech had hot sauce in her desk which he proceeded to spray over the walls. The sheriff office was called and John apprehended the patient, and I got to know him.

"Hey John, what is going on?" I asked.

"This is for you, man. We're honoring all of our staff who are here today fighting this pandemic," he said.

There were perhaps a hundred officers and firemen lined up along the sidewalk cheering nurses, doctors and staff as we were coming to start our shift or leaving to go home. There were hand-written signs of appreciation for our efforts during the pandemic.

"This is so cool," I told John. "We should be honoring you too," I said.

I have been working in a medical center for 40 years and have never seen anything like this. It was gratifying to see that these officers were thanking us.

*

In late August of 2020, on the South Lawn of the White House, President Donald Trump accepted the Republican Party's nomination for President. The Party organizers invited nurses and first responders on the front line tending to patients infected with COVID-19. During his speech, President Trump asked that these individuals stand and accept his "profound thanks and gratitude" for their work. He then remarked that the US developed the largest system for COVID-19 testing anywhere in the world. But what he and other leaders from both parties have largely failed to recognize was the effort needed to develop laboratory tests for the coronavirus, and more importantly, the personal health risk these laboratory staff take in collecting samples and performing testing.

"The risks you face are equal to what your colleagues on the wards face," I said to Rada one day, "because we are in direct contact with them and their body fluids."

"It is the involuntary flinches that I fear most," Rada replied. "Sometimes the needle gets pulled out of the vein. That is when my job is the most dangerous."

*

Despite following all precautions and wearing personal protective equipment at all times when drawing blood, Rada contracted COVID. She entered a room of a patient who didn't have symptoms and who the medical staff did not suspect that the patient was infected with COVID. Some of the staff attending her were themselves not properly protected with N95 masks. It was unclear how Rada contracted the virus. The hospital did not initially provide face shields, and it is possible that a cough aerosol from an infected patient entered Rada's fluid within her eyes.

Once she developed symptoms, Rada checked in to the emergency room at a hospital near her home. She was well aware of the symptoms of having collected blood from many COVID-19 patients. I got a call from her mother saying that Rada was very sick and in the hospital's intensive care unit. I was helpless to help her. Even as a healthcare worker, I was not able to visit her in the ICU. Her major medical problem was difficulty in breathing and was put on a ventilator. Word got out in the laboratory that Rada was sick with COVID-19. I gathered my group and asked that we prayed for her recovery. Cards and flowers were delivered to her hospital bed

*

On the next day, we got word that Rada passed. Her nurses told her that Rada fought hard to live. But in the end, she was all alone when she died. She was only 29 years old. She was not able to have an in-personal funeral. A ceremony was held via a teleconference. In all my years in the clinical laboratory, Rada was the only one to die from an occupational-related infection or injury. With permission from my Department head, we named the phlebotomy station at our hospital in her honor. In addition, I had a patch made with a note saying, "Ask me about Rada." This patch was given to all of our phlebotomists to sew onto the sleeve of their lab coat. Everybody was honored to wear this tribute to her.

*

Hospitals, medical centers and healthcare workers who provide care to patient who have contracted a highly contagious disease exercise policies that greatly minimize the possibility of infection to themselves and other. Patients are isolated into special units where there is positive or negative pressure ventilation that divert airflow away from the external environment and to special filters that trap viral-contaminated air. Healthcare workers entering these rooms must don disposable personal protective equipment (PPE) which include use of gowns, gloves, ventilators, and shields. For some isolation units, often there is an "anteroom," a separate room between the corridor and the room itself. This is where nurses, doctors, respiratory therapists, phlebotomists, etc. can put on their PPE before entering the patient room, and remove them for discard before leaving the area entirely. During the different waves of COIVID-19 infections, the number of cases have exceed the number of isolation rooms available, and these additional precautions were not always available. This increased the risk of transmission to healthcare workers, such as what occurred to Rada. False negative coronavirus test results may also contribute to unexpected transmission of the virus to caregivers. While there have been many healthcare workers that have become infected by treating COVID-19 patients, the majority of the cases are acquired through community spread. Healthcare workers are the most knowledgeable about routes of infections, and can take the necessary precautions within their day-to-day contacts outside work to minimize risk of transmission.

The Bubble

The great COVID-19 pandemic disrupted the lives of everyone on the planet. The hardest hit countries suspended most non-essential work activities for many months. For the safety of the athletes, coaches, and spectators, professional and amateur sports such as basketball, baseball, soccer, hockey, golf, and tennis, were suspended during the early months of the pandemic. It was fortunate that the professional and college football seasons had ended just prior to the outbreak and their 2019 season was saved. Gradually, these sports opened up their seasons under various conditions to minimize risk of infection by the coronavirus. Many of the sport's stars have opted out of participating in post-COVID-19 events like Buster Posey of Baseball's San Francisco Giants and Rafael Nadal of men's tennis. Some professional golfers like Brooks Koepka, opted out of some of the early PGA events, but have resumed their competitions.

*

I received a call from Diane Carter, a senior executive of a company who was familiar with my work in laboratory medicine over the past several years. She told me that one of the professional sport leagues was planning on limited resumption of their season and they needed somebody from the clinical laboratory who could advise them about testing for COVID-19. She wanted to know if I was interested in helping them. I advised Diane that I was neither a virologist nor an epidemiologist, and therefore I could not help them with the basic science of coronavirus infections or how virus surveillance and contact tracing is performed. She assured me that there were other experts on the panel that had been engaged in those types of discussions. What they wanted was advice on the best approach for testing the presence of the virus, and the human antibodies that the virus produces. As I was engaged in these very same discussions with our medical staff regarding COVID-19 testing for our hospital and outpatient clinics, I thought that I might qualify. But as I am not a microbiology laboratory or molecular diagnostics laboratory director, I question if there might be anybody else more qualified.

"I thought of you because not only are you versed with the clinical laboratory practice, but through your translational research program, you had broad knowledge of the in vitro diagnostics industry," Diane said. This was true. Over the years, I have worked with all of the major diagnostic companies in performing clinical trials to get their commercial laboratory tests approved by the FDA, and adopted for clinical practice in hospital laboratories such as ours. Diane has been with several of these companies, and I had worked with her in the past. "They are going to need an unbiased review of the available commercial tests that best suits their current need."

"Why did they contact your company first?" I asked Diane.

"Our testing platform is one of the options they are considering. But I told them that we were just one of the many different approaches that can be taken towards COVID-19 testing, and my opinions are biased towards our products. I told them that what they needed was somebody who is not associated with any one company and could give them an honest assessment of their plans, so I thought of you."

I was extremely flattered that Diane thought of me for the job. Then I thought that maybe everybody else she tried to contact turned her down. I was even more impressed that the executive from the league didn't just take testing for granted and knew that they need to fully vet the various choices available. I indicated my interest in the project and Diane gave me the email and telephone number of Lamar McMichael, an attorney and vice president for the league. I sent an email indicating my interest in participating, and we set up a call for later that same evening. It was 10:00 pm on the East Coast. *This is going to move fast*, I thought to myself.

"Ownership and the players' union have agreed to resume our season. There will be a limited number of games prior to a multi-team playoff. All the games will take place in one city, with players, coaches, and management of each team being sequestered among themselves. Players who agree to our stipulation will not be allowed to interact with anybody outside of their "bubble." There will be no fans attending. All the games will be televised nationally."

*

The last time the U.S. suspended some of its major sports activities was in the week following the 9/11 attack in 2001. Professional hockey, basketball and football hadn't started its season yet, and Major league baseball resumed its season one week later. Prior to 9/11, the previous disruption of sports occurred nearly 80 years during the Second World War. Many of the college football teams, more popular than professional football, stopped playing for the duration of the war. Motorcycle and automobile racing was suspended because the rubber and gasoline was needed for the war effort. Baseball continued its season but without many of the game's biggest stars. This led in part to the formation of an All-American Girl Baseball League was formed during the war by Chicago Cub's owner William Wrigley. Outside the US, the English Football Association (soccer) canceled the remainder of the 1939 season after Germany invaded Poland. However, soccer games did resume during the war but with limited attendance by fans. It was argued then that spectator sports was good for the morale of the citizenship. Both the 1940 and 1944 Summer and Winter Olympics were cancelled during World War II. Interestingly, except for England, the host countries for these games were supposed to be Japan, Germany, and Italy, members of the defeated

Axis Powers.

During the 2020 COVID pandemic, several important sporting events were cancelled including the NCAA Basketball tournament (aka, "March Madness"), the College World Series (Baseball), Wimbledon Tennis Championship, and the British Open Golf Tournament. These events had been held continuously since the end of World War II. The absence of sports damaged the sports betting industry, especially March Madness. Cities that are heavily involved with gaming, for example Las Vegas, lost billions of dollars in gambling revenue.

*

Lamar told me of the plan the league has for resuming the season and the protocol for protecting the players who agreed to participate, coaches, and their team's personnel. Air travel was the initial concern, as individuals are exposed to fellow passengers in a closed environment for many hours at a time. However, most of this fear was unfounded as the circulation within an airplane is good. A bigger concern is local transportation within buses, trains, and taxis where the contact with fellow passengers and drivers and the air ventilation is not controlled. The importance of wearing masks and practicing social distancing whenever possible, were stressed. Once assembled in the city selected for all of the games, everyone must quarantine and pass two COVID tests before they are released into their respective bubble. Individuals who test positive are quarantined for at least 14 days. They were not allowed to enter another player's room or socialize with other players or friends staying at a different hotel. All food is provided by the team within the team's bubble. Lamar indicated that the league did hire some of the best chefs that they could find.

"In essence, they are prisoners of their environment," I commented to Lamar.

"This is not like opening up a factory for employees that makes widgets. This activity will be highly scrutinized by the media and general public. Any mistake will be magnified. We are taking a big chance on the health of these athletes," Lamar said.

"The good news, is that they are all incredibly healthy and physically fit, with little or no co-morbidities. If they were to get infected, their mortality is extremely unlikely," I stated.

Lamar estimated that thousands of individuals will need to be tested each day during the restarted season, with results made available to the team physicians on the following morning. It was determined that logistically, this could only be achieved if testing is performed locally. We discussed the possibility of academic versus commercial laboratories. I made some inquiries about the potential for testing among my colleagues at some of the state's most prominent medical centers. Unfortunately, they did not have the personnel, especially during the night shift to handle such a large influx of samples. Qualified technologists are difficult to hire on short notice because of the required qualifications and training. Moreover, at these hospitals, their priority was testing their own patients and healthcare workers.

Another issue was reagent supply. At my hospital, we used a mixture of several different testing platforms because no single manufacturer could promise enough reagents to handle our daily testing needs. If there was an interruption in the supply of test kits, the remainder of the season could be in jeopardy. In the end, the league selected a reference laboratory that had the experience and capacity to perform the work. I was asked to review the qualifications of the laboratory in terms of equipment, personnel, and competency of their tests. In our profession, all certified laboratories must undergo "proficiency testing," a comparison of tests results between laboratories using the same sample. In this situation, I sent a mix of nasopharyngeal swabs from patients that we already tested for COVID-19 to the commercial testing lab. I asked them to provide me raw data results to compare against ours. When a test is positive for coronavirus using PCR, the number of cycles required for test signal to cross the cycle threshold (CT) is recorded. The lower the number of cycles, the higher the viral load count. The result is considered negative when the threshold signal is not reached after 40 cycles. In comparing a couple of dozen samples, we saw a 100% concordance of positive versus negative samples, and excellent agreements of the cycle number for positive samples. I also had the reference laboratory send data on the analytical sensitivity of their testing platform. This was a major issue to Lamar.

"If there is any hint of a positive result, we need to take preventative action. We cannot afford any errors," he said.

I fully agreed with the plan and thought that the lab they selected could do as good of a job as anyone and still meet the turnaround time needs. I then had a deeper, philosophical discussion with Lamar. I knew it was a little out of why they hired me, but I wanted to know where they might go with this.

"In the unlikely event that a player contracts COVID-19, is hospitalized, and subsequently dies, what will the league do?" I asked.

"Legally, all of the players have signed a contract indicating that they are accepting the risks for resuming their season. Of course, all medical expenses will be covered by us." Lamar commented. "Their medical information would be protected by privacy laws."

"You know that is not what I meant. I am talking about ethically. Will the team drop out of competition? Will the league terminate the season? I could see that this would be a public relations nightmare. What do you say to the surviving family?" I knew I didn't have the right to ask these questions, but I believed I had a rapport with Lamar and he would be honest about what they are thinking.

"The closest thing we have in history to this is the Pat Tillman story," Lamar pointed out.

Tillman played the position of safety for the Arizona

Cardinals.   A few months after the 9/11 attacks, he suspended his football career with the NFL and his $3.6 million contract to enlist into the Army with his brother in June 2012. After basic training, he was deployed in Iraq and then Afghanistan. In April, 2004, Tillman was accidently shot three times in the head by friendly fire in April 2004. The American forces heard gunshots that were mistakenly thought to have originated from the enemy. Tillman died that day.

"Pat Tillman's sacrifice is revered by the nation today. I think if one of our players died of COVID, we would suspend the season for a week in honor of our fallen colleague. Depending on how his family reacted, but we would state that he loved the game, and would want his teammates and opponents to continue. Our league is a very tight knit group, with most of the players on very friendly terms with the others," Lamar continued. "I can imagine that we would retire this player's jersey from his team and possibly the league." Lamar may have been referring to Major League Baseball's 1997 retirement of Jackie Robinson's uniform number 42 from all major league teams. Robinson was the first African American to play in the Major Leagues.

*

The first few days of testing was conducted on team staff, before the players arrived. When the first set of results came back, there was some concerns. Some of the individuals tested had a borderline positive result that turned negative on the next day and vice versa. The interpretation of this result was not clear.

"All laboratory tests have some degree of uncertainty when results fall near the threshold," I told Lamar. "That is because all lab tests have variabilities. It is one of the reasons that repeating borderline samples is a good idea. It is also a prudent to obtain a fresh sample and to test again."

Lamar was reassured that their testing policies were sound.

"When it comes to the analysis for coronavirus, there is an additional issue," I said. "There can be a positive result due to the shedding of the virus from someone who was infected at some distant point in the past. This does not necessarily mean that they are actively infected or more importantly, *actively infectious*. One thing you can try to do in these borderline cases, is to test for COVID-19 antibodies. A positive result would suggest a past infection. You can also send the nasopharyngeal swab for sequencing of the entire RNA virus."

"How does that help?" Lamar asked.

"If there are non-viable remnant viral particles present, the sample will be able to be sequenced," I said. "But that is not done in clinical laboratories, so testing is largely not available."

In the end, these individuals were quarantined as the league could not take any chances. The league resumed its season without incident. Nobody suffered from a significant illness. Television ratings for the events were excellent. Professional sports can claim that they have boosted the morale of the general public while stimulating the economy at the same time.

*

After a several month of hiatus, professional sports slowly resumed. One of the first events took place on May 24th when Tiger Woods teamed up with Peyton Manning and Phil Mickelson joined Tom Brady for a televised charity golf challenge. Sports fans welcomed the diversion from the mundane shelter-in-place existence and watching reruns of past sporting events. Since golf is played outdoors and there is no physical contact between participants, it was an ideal game to re-open. The sport was not without issues, however, as several golfers including Nick Watney learned that he contracted COVID-19 after playing in the first round of the RBC Heritage tournament in June and immediately withdrew. Major League Baseball also suffered from COVID-19 infections among players and coaches. As of the end of July, more than half of the active players on the Miami Marlins team and 2 coaches contracted COVID and were placed on quarantine. They were replaced with minor league players and the team proceeded to go on a winning streak and made it to the postseason. FC Dallas of Major League Soccer withdrew from the championship tournament after 10 players and one coach tested positive. Novak Djokovic, the top ranked player in men's tennis, and his wife tested positive for COVID-19 but both were asymptomatic. He has subsequently tested negative and has participated in the U.S. Open. The 2020 Olympics in Tokyo have been rescheduled for 2021. Many Division I College Football schools and conferences have cancelled, postponed, or reduced their 2020 schedule. Nick Sabin, Head

Coach of the Alabama Football team has contracted COVID. This was a temporary setback as the team later won the National Championship. In the NFL, 24 individuals including 11 players of the Tennessee Titans tested positive and games were postponed. The Titans went on to soundly defeat the Buffalo Bills when their season resumed. The Denver Broncos played their game against the New Orleans Saints without any of their quarterbacks, as Jeff Driskel tested positive and interacted with Drew Lock, Brett Rypien, and Blake Bortles without wearing a mask and all were not allowed to play. Needless to say, the team was soundly defeated.

There have been deaths of professional sports figures while they were engaged in a competitive season. In 2002, Darryl Kile a pitcher for the St. Louis Cardinals died of a heart attack and was found dead in his hotel room. The game between them and the Chicago Cubs was postponed on that day. Seven years later, Nicholas Adenhart, a pitcher for the Anaheim Angels, died in a car crash a few hours after pitching in a game. At Arizona State University in Tempe, there is a larger-than-life statue of Pat Tillman at the school's Sun Devil Stadium and another in Glendale, Arizona, where the Cardinals play. His number 42 and number 40 jerseys that he wore in college and in the NFL have been retired.

When the shortened seasons were completed for the various team and individual sports, it was clear that the "bubble" concept of restricting gatherings was more successful than asking each athlete to adhere to guidelines on a voluntary basis. These are young vibrant men and women who have more than the usual sense of "invincibility" for people in this age bracket. Moreover, most are multi-millionaires who are used to getting what they want.

Socialization, i.e., partying with friends and acquaintances, are a major source of recreation for these athletes. So to prohibit this activity outside of their social bubble was a perceived hardship. Then again, there is little sympathy by the general public, many who were sheltered-in-place at the expense of earning a living.

In August of 2020, the National Football League received positive test results from 77 of its players at the same time from one laboratory. The original samples were repeated and found to be negative. A second sample collected from these players were also all negative. Based on this, the laboratory declared that the original tests were falsely positive. This created quite a havoc among players and teams alike. The tested samples were accidentally contaminated by RNA from an unknown source. Because molecular tests require amplification of nucleic acid material, there are a number of ways samples can become contaminated. Usually, the laboratory has procedural and environmental controls to prevent this from occurring. However, there can be transmission of viral nucleic acids from aerosolization of fluids, human handling of samples, and inadequate cleansing of instruments and surfaces.

My "what if" discussions with the league was fictitious. To date, there have been no deaths of a professional athlete due to COVID. Testing continues to be the key in resuming sports competitions.

With the release of the COVID-19 vaccine, it was tempting for professional athletes and management staff to want to receive it ahead of healthcare workers and other essential personnel. To their credit, they did not exercised their wealth and influence to "jump their players in front of the line." That is, they were given the same priority as other citizens.

The March of Quarters

****

In September of 1937, President Franklin D. Roosevelt announced the creation of the National Foundation for Infantile Paralysis. At the time infections by poliomyelitis was the leading cause of childhood disability, with over 7 cases per 100,000 of the American population. FDR himself was a victim of polio, although he did not become paralyzed until he reached 39 years of age. The singer and Hollywood film star, Eddie Cantor, was involved with raising money for this Foundation by hosting balls each year on FDR's birthday. The National Foundation was incorporated in January of the following year. Cantor coined the fund-raising ads on the radio as "The March of Quarters." Mail containing quarters were sent to the White House months later and by the date of FDR's birthday, the Foundation had raised $268,000 (equivalent to over $1.8 million in today's dollars).

*

During this period, Jonas Rosenberg was attending medical school at New York University, School of Medicine. NYU was one of the few medical schools on the East Coast that didn't discriminate against Jewish applicants. He was the son of immigrants who came to the U.S. in the early 1920s from a small village in Romania. While in middle school, his father contracted the Spanish Flu and tragically died shortly thereafter. Jonas had to work after school in New York City's garment district as an aide. This motivated Jonas for a better life. He was a brilliant student, skipping grades in high school and earned a Bachelor's degree in chemistry at the age of 19. After graduating medical school, Dr. Rosenberg began working at the University of Michigan, where he helped develop a vaccine to influenza. *This is for you Pop,* he thought to himself.

Two years after the end of World War II, Dr. Rosenberg joined the faculty of the University of Pittsburgh School of Medicine. He received funds from the National Foundation for Infantile Paralysis as well as the National Institute of Health, and began his work on developing a polio vaccine.

*

Four-year old Ronald Madison, an only child, came home from his daycare center with a sore throat and fever. He also complained to his mother, Roberta, of neck pain. His mother was a nurse at the local hospital, took some days off from work and kept Ronald home for the remainder of the week. Her husband was a marine fighting in the Korean War. Over the weekend, Ronald developed progressive weakness in his joints and legs. Roberta feared the worse, so she took him to see his doctor, who diagnosed him as having a polio infection.

"There is not much we can do. Keep him comfortable and hope for the best," his doctor said.

Roberta started crying. She had seen many children in her hospital with the disease and she knew it could be fatal. Ronald was not visibly upset and tried to calm her down. "Don't worry, Mommy. I will be fine. I know I will get better." But the boy did not improve and over the course of the next few months, his right leg began to atrophy. He could no longer walk without assistance. The family got a wheelchair from the hospital and Roberta fitted him with crutches. After some instruction, the now five-year old child was doing well. "See, Mommy? I can get around and don't need anybody's help." Roberta couldn't believe the positive attitude that her son was taking. He never complained or ask why this happened to him. He was content to occupy himself with his dog, play with his Tonka toy trucks, and listen to the Hoody Doody show on the radio.

*

That same year, after several years of work, Dr. Rosenberg announced the launch of a clinical trial for his experimental polio vaccine. Previous trials using weakened virus had failed. Instead, he used a virus that had been rendered biologically inactive. In his initial studies, he inoculated several dozen children. Confident of its safety and efficacy to give to others, and against all medical ethics, Dr. Rosenberg injected his own children early in the process. With no medical complications observed in his pilot studies, he received additional funding to use his vaccine on a mass basis. It was a highly publicized activity that attracted countless number of contributors to the March of Quarters. It took thousands of physicians, healthcare workers, school personnel and volunteers to educate and administer the vaccine to the nation's children.

In April 1955, it was announced that the vaccine was safe. Due to the scale of this program, and the fact that FDR suffered from polio, Dr. Rosenberg became an international celebrity. He received many awards, honorary university degrees, met heads of state, and he received invitations to give keynote speeches. Jonas and his research team did not seek a patent for his polio vaccine. This philanthropic gesture greatly accelerated the distribution of the polio vaccine to the US and the entire world.

However, Jonas was not happy about the demands of a public figure. It took time away from his research. "I am more interested in gaining the respect of my peers than the general public," he once said to his wife. At the age of

41, he was at the prime of his intellectual capabilities. At least, he didn't have paparazzi to deal with. His fame did enable funding for the creation of the Rosenberg Institute for Biological Studies in 1963 and headquartered in La Jolla, California. Over the ensuing decades, he and his fellow scientists pioneered many areas of modern science and medicine. One of the resident scientists, Roger Guillemin, received the Nobel Prize for Medicine in 1977, for his work on neurohormones.

*

A few years before the availability of the polio vaccines, John Sutter, one of the executive directors for the March of Quarters came up with a fundraising idea. "I want to find a boy or girl afflicted with polio and make him a poster child," he said to other executives in a board room meeting.

Dr. Jonas Rosenberg was in attendance and asked, "What is a poster boy?"

"We would put the child on our advertisements stating that the money to support the March of Quarters would help these unfortunate children who got sick through no fault of their own. We are appealing to emotional concerns of parents."

"Has this type of advertisement ever been done before?" Dr. Silvia Mitchell, a pediatrician and board member asked.

"No, this is a new idea that was suggested to me by my teenage daughter," John said. "If this works, we could select a different child every year."

"I know a 5-year old boy who could be the first child," Dr. Mitchell said. "One of my nurses has a child who has polio. She is a widow as her husband was killed in action in Korea while serving our country and she is raising him alone. I have gotten to know Ronnie. He is a happy child and has accepted his disability. I think he would be perfect."

Roberta agreed to allow Ronnie to be photographed along with Jonas Rosenberg. The poster showed the boy with a very determined face, denoting that this disease was not going to stop him from achieving his goals in life. At that time, Dr. Rosenberg was not yet a celebrity. Over the ensuing years, other boys and girls were selected as the poster child for the Foundation. They posed with many of the Hollywood actors, singers, sports celebrities, and politicians of the day such including Marilyn Monroe, Elvis Presley, Joe DiMaggio, and President John F Kennedy. After the vaccine was released, these children became sort of celebrities themselves. During the year, Ronnie embraced his role as a spokesperson for the Institute. When it was over, he returned to a quiet life with his mother and friends.

*

Carolina Carinko was born in 1955, a few weeks before Dr. Rosenberg's announcement of an effective vaccine for polio. Carolina lived in the same Romanian village that Dr. Rosenberg's parents were from. Ten years into the polio vaccine era, the village's leadership invited Jonas Rosenberg and his mother to celebrate their achievements. Young Carolina got to meet the good doctor during their visit. Inspired by this meeting, Carolina devoted herself to science. She excelled in school and received a scholarship to the Romanian Institute of Science and Technology, where she earned a doctoral degree in immunology. After several postdoctoral appointments in Romania and the U.S., she became an Assistant Professor at the University of Pennsylvania. Her work involved using messenger RNA (mRNA) to produce therapeutic proteins.

*

At the General Hospital, my chemistry laboratory supervisor was Jean Brach. Jean was born in Guatemala and was a fraternal twin. She and her brother John became scientists. John married Elizabeth Blackman, a fellow scholar originally from Australia. Dr. Blackman pioneered work on telomeres, an important enzyme involved with aging. For this work, she shared the Nobel Prize in Physiology or Medicine in 2009. The award ceremony is given each year in Stockholm. I asked Jean if she was going to attend her sister-in-law's once-in-a-lifetime award event. While she had plenty of vacation time available to her, she told me that wanted to stay at home and continue her important work managing our clinical laboratory staff. She was that kind of person. In 2015, Dr. Blackman left the University and became the President at the Rosenberg Institute for Biological Sciences, a post she held for 2 years before her retirement.

*

Ronnie became a US Post Office worker in Seattle, Washington for 25 years before his retirement. He is still married to his high school sweetheart. They have 3 children and 9 grandchildren. In the summer of 2020, he contracted a SARS-CoV-2 infection. Ronnie suffered from significant breathing problems and was hospitalized for 30 days. He was treated with Remdesivir and Regeneron antibodies which was effective, and he survived. His wife and family were not able to see him while he was in the hospital. He was able to text and occasionally phone his family telling them he loved them and that he was going to survive. His wife, watching new reports of the horrendous death rates in their area due to COVID-19, was not so sure. On the day of his discharge, the nurses and doctors lined up the hallway as he was wheeled-chaired out of the hospital. When he emerged outside to an atypically cloudless Seattle day, his son was playing the Beatles' song, *Here Comes the Sun*. There were tears of joy streaming from the faces of his family members.

Months later, Ronnie donated some of his plasma containing COVID-19 antibodies for use in treating other COVID-19 infected patients.

*

In the early 1990s, Dr. Carolina Carinko's research at U Penn was struggling. Using mRNA, her idea was to induce human cells to produce foreign proteins. Deoxyribonucleic acid or DNA resides in the body's nucleus, and is the blueprint for producing all of the proteins needed for an organism to live and thrive. The cell's protein-producing mechanism resides within the cytoplasm. mRNA is a shorter piece that is transferred from the nucleus to the cytoplasm, and contains the recipe for the cell to produce a specific protein needed for the organism's existence. Dr. Carinko's idea was to inject a synthetic form of mRNA that contained a specific sequence that encode the amino acids needed to produce a foreign viral protein into human cells, in hopes of fooling it to produce the viral protein. Once that new viral protein is produced and circulating in the body, the plan was that person's immune system would recognize it as foreign and raise antibodies against it. The key to the success of this research was for the human cell to produce the foreign protein only temporarily. Therefore, she needed to modify the structure of the nucleic acid bases within the mRNA, so that it would be recognized by the host immune system as foreign and eventually destroy it. If the host destroys the mRNA too soon, however, it won't have a chance to do to its job.

Dr. Carinko spent years of research trying to find how to appropriately modify the mRNA. In the meantime, her research funding began to diminish. She wrote numerous grants to the National Institute of Health on her concept but did not have enough preliminary data to show that her theory could work. With no funding, Dr. Carinko was demoted academically and her research lab was on the verge of being dismantled by her Department. Noticing that she was on the verge of a nervous breakdown, a colleague, Dr. Drake Weinberg, came into her office.

"Carolina, you look really depressed. Is there something wrong? he asked.

"Everything is collapsing around me. I just got another bad score on my NIH grant, and it will not get funded. My husband traveled home to see his ailing mother and immigration is giving him a hard time with his visa. And now, my doctor thinks I may have a tumor in my breast. I don't know if I can stand it anymore," Dr. Carinko said.

"Last week, our department chair has asked me to review your grant. He is very supportive of you but he has to decide if he can justify keeping you here without sustained funding. I think the science has a lot of potential. The key now is to find just the right synthetic nucleic base that can temporarily escape recognition by the human immune system. I think I have an idea that you can try," Drake said.

"I would love to try something new. What did you have in mind?"

This conversation with Dr. Weinberg invigorated Caroline. She also thought back about her meeting as a child with Jonas Rosenberg, and that he would not quit to achieve his goals. She heard that Dr. Rosenberg had passed away just a few months earlier. With Drake's help, they determined that rather than using synthetic mRNA, they only needed to modify uracil, just one of mRNA's four bases. This change allowed the mRNA to survive long enough for protein transcription before it is degraded by the human body.

Their scientific discovery went largely unnoticed for many years. Eventually other scientists saw the potential of this technology to produce the next generation of vaccines.

They acquired the rights to Dr. Carinko's patents and two companies were formed, BioNTech and Moderna. When the COVID-19 pandemic hit Wuhan. China in December of 2019, these two companies began work on a vaccine using the mRNA technology.

Within a few months after the onset of the pandemic, Moderna and BioNTech in collaboration with Pfizer, conducted clinical trials to determine the efficacy and safety of their mRNA coronavirus vaccine. The mRNA vaccine stimulates the host to produce the critically important spike protein of SARS-CoV-2. In December 2020, just one year after the pandemic, both companies received FDA clearance under the Emergency Use Authorization. Healthcare workers and first responders were among the first to receive the vaccine.

Despite the efficacy and safety profile of the new vaccines, much of the general public was reluctant to accept use of the vaccine to COVID-19. The March of Quarters underwent a campaign to educate the public. They reached out to Elizabeth Blackman to come out of retirement and help with the educational effort. The March of Quarters located Ronnie Madison and Dr. Blackman spoke with the former poster child. He told her that he was a COVID-19 survivor and was happy to participate. The pair filmed social media videos to boost the importance of taking the vaccine. The video was posted onto the internet.

"Hello, my name is Ronnie Madison and this is a public service announcement. I have survived two of the world's most deadly viral diseases of the last 100 years. There were no vaccines available to me for either disease at the time of my illnesses. Please don't let COVID-19 happen to you."

"And my name is Elizabeth Blackman. I am the former President of the Rosenberg Institute. Our Institute founder, Dr. Jonas Rosenberg, developed the first vaccine for polio and today, it has largely been eradicated."

The camera panned back to show both Ronnie and Elizabeth. "If we are to eradicate COVID-19, everybody needs to do their part in fighting this killer," Elizabeth said. "Take the vaccine when it is offered to you. Protect yourself and your loved ones," Ronnie said. "Let there be sunny days ahead into our lives." This message meant to fight against a real virus went viral.

*

This story has been fictionalized but is largely based on true events. Most individuals who were born before 1950 will know the devastated effects of polio, and the invaluable contributions of Jonas Salk and the polio vaccine. In light of the COVID-19 pandemic, it was important to retell this tale to a younger audience who have no direct experience with the polio virus. While the two current COVID-19 vaccines are fundamentally different from the one Salk developed, the overall objectives of obtaining mass human immunity are identical.

The first March of Dimes poster child was Donald Anderson from Prineville, Oregon, who contracted polio at the age of 6 and became the first March of Dimes poster child in 1946. He was born too soon to benefit from the vaccine, but his participation help raised the money that was needed. Donald worked for the US Postal Office, had 4 children and 7 grandchildren before he died at the age of 73 in 2014. With polio largely eradicated, the mission of the March of Dimes has shifted to other pediatric problems, including research on the cause and prevention of premature births.

Katalin Karikó and Drew Weissman were Professors at the University of Pennsylvania when they discovered pseudouridine as a nucleoside modification that suppressed the immunogencity of RNA. This ultimately enabled the production and release of the COVID-19 vaccine by Pfizer/BioNTech and Moderna in record time. Shortly after these vaccines were approved, AstraZeneca received approval for their vaccine, which involves injection of a modified and harmless version of the common cold.

It should be noted that Jonas Salk's mother was from Minsk of what is now Belarus, and Katalin Karikó was from a small town in Hungary. Dr. Salk died in 1995, and the two likely never met.

Elizabeth Blackburn was not involved with Donald Anderson's COVID-19 vaccine campaign. Her sister-in-law, Jean Branch was the senior supervisor for my hospital's core laboratory for many years. She passed away in 2020 following an illness unrelated to COVID-19. We will dedicate part of our lab in her honor.

On March 11, 2021, four of the five former Presidents of the United States (Jimmy Carter, Bill Clinton, George W. Bush, and Barack Obama) and their wives made a public service announcement promoting the citizenship to take one of the vaccines available when their turn is up. This follows the tradition that was first started by the March of Dimes for the polio vaccine over 60 years earlier. Only Donald Trump declined the appear.

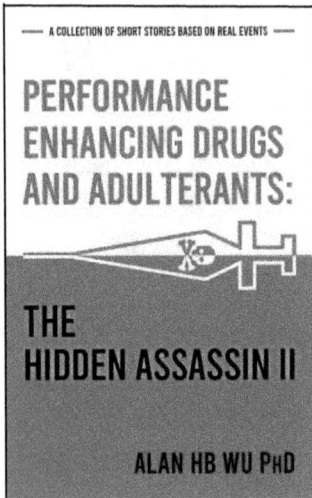

Urine Luck

****

In high school there are the preppies, the jocks, the drama queens, the nerds, and the potheads. Jaco Jamison was clearly in the last category. He spent much time in the bathroom smoking cigarettes or an occasional joint before attending class. "I'm never going to need to know this shit," he told his mother. His mother knew that he wasn't dumb, just unmotivated. His car reeked of cigarette and marijuana smoke. Butts and crumpled rolling papers crammed the dashboard ashtray. He kept his windows closed for fear that the smell would reveal him to the school narcs, but everyone knew what he was up to anyway and didn't care.

Jaco was always good with cars and motorcycles. The kids brought all their mechanical problems to him. So when Jaco left high school, his classmates were not surprised that he was able to land a steady job as a garage man at the city's bus depot. By then, he was smoking dope regularly, yet it didn't interfere with his job. He became a master at concealing his drug use from his superiors. He worked at the bus depot garage for eight years and they eventually transferred him to driving the city's bus. This was easier than working on engines. The promotion, however, required him as well as other drivers, to undergo routine urine drug and alcohol testing.

Jaco did not want to lose his new job by failing a urine test; he needed the money to support his drug lifestyle. He was able to stop smoking hash for a month while he started his new job. In the meantime, he learned all he could about drug testing policies and procedures so he could beat them. If he had studied this much in high school, he could have been a lawyer by now. One of the first things he found out was that you can buy at-home urine drug testing kits on the Internet. These tests were similar to the lab-based test his employer used. Although purchasing these kits on a regular basis became expensive, it was better than losing his job with a positive drug test. The bus company always scheduled their drug test quarterly. Since they did not do them randomly, Jaco's plan was to abstain from smoking five days prior to the appointment. He tested his own urine using the kit just to be sure.

"If I test positive, I'll just call in sick that day," he told his unemployed co-druggie roommate. This plan worked for several years. But he wanted more. He believed he could beat the system without even having to stop smoking before the test.

Why should I cease my enjoyment four times a year? he thought. His new plan was to drink copious amounts of water to dilute his urine just prior to self-testing. Jaco learned that in order for his urine to come out positive, the amount of drug in the urine had to exceed the test's threshold. He had this down to a science; he knew exactly how much he could smoke and how much water he needed to drink to get below the test cutoff. Besides, he always owned the 'I am sick today' excuse as his get out-of-jail card. This worked for years. He knew he was playing with fire, but he didn't want to get off pot.

*

Calvin was in the nerd set in high school. His parents emigrated from Taiwan when he was two years old. He did well in math and made friends through the science club. He was small for his age having reached puberty later than the other boys. He was shy around girls at school; most of them were bigger than he was. While they went to the same school, Jaco and Calvin didn't know each other. Their only encounter was when Calvin was a freshman and Jaco was in his fifth year of high school. Calvin desperately had to pee before algebra. Not knowing the unofficial bathroom rules, he went into the smoker's john. Jaco and his friends saw the little kid, pushed him against a stall, and told Calvin to beat it. After that encounter, Calvin said to himself, *someday I'm going to stand up to those guys.*

Calvin went to college, majoring in chemistry. Science was easy for him, and he was eager to learn. Right out of college, he landed a job in my toxicology laboratory. We were doing workplace drug testing at the time. Calvin's job was to process the hundreds of urine samples each day and load them into the instruments for testing. He felt overqualified for this work, but he had to start somewhere. The worst part of the job was the awful smell. Sometimes, he would spill some urine onto his clothes, shoes, and socks. Fortunately, we had a shower in the lab and he kept extra clothes on hand. I recognized that Calvin had a keen eye for details, and I wanted him to advance.

After a few years, I asked Calvin, "Why don't you go back to school and earn your master's degree in forensic science, which includes those involved with workplace drug testing? Then we can have you do more interesting jobs that suit your talents." With that encouragement, Calvin enrolled in night school while keeping his day job working for me. When Calvin finished two years later, I promoted him to certifying scientist. His new job was to look at toxicology data and verify their results. By now, he was no longer the shy introverted person he'd been when he was young. Calvin met a girl, married, and together they had a daughter named Jenny.

*

Jaco's urine sample was routinely sent to the lab for testing. Unknowingly, Calvin had been involved with Jaco's urine testing for years. The samples were identified by number only. Jaco's samples were simply labeled as #32449. In going through his daily records, Calvin noticed that one sample reported as negative was just below the cutoff for THC. THC is tetrahydrocannabinol, the active ingredient of marijuana. This sample also contained a low level of creatinine. While creatinine is a normal component of urine, low values indicate urine dilution by higher than normal fluid intake. Calvin went back into the records and found that #32449 consistently produced these results. He came to my office to show me what he had discovered.

I told him, "Some people have other drugs or constituents in their urine that may trigger a false reaction to the THC test. Our cutoffs differentiate between what is truly positive from interferents. Besides, people can have small amounts of marijuana in their urine due to passive exposure. Calvin, you wouldn't want us to report a positive result just because someone was at a rock concert and exposed to others who were smoking, would you?"

"I guess not," he said. But Calvin wasn't satisfied. How could #32449 be at a rock concert each time he was drug tested? Although he knew he could get in trouble for this, Calvin kept one of #32449's urine samples aside in the freezer. He removed it one day when I was away. Opening the cup, he let it stand at room temperature to let some of the water evaporate. When this concentrated urine was retested, it came out positive. *I've have my eye on you #32449*, he said to himself, and then discarded the cup.

Jaco's driving record was without incident. This

eventually landed him a job driving kids at his old high school. They were mostly freshmen and sophomores who didn't have drivers' licenses yet or whose parents couldn't afford cars for them. He was ten years older than most of them and they treated him like he was Fonzie from Happy Days; the cool driver dude. He still had to undergo regular drug testing and he still was participant #32449. By this time, he'd gotten tired of drinking excess fluids prior to his tests and learned about adulteration products. He purchased Urine Luck from the Internet in hopes of taking his deception to the next level. Urine Luck was a commercially available urine drug-testing adulterant. It consisted of a vial containing one ounce of a yellow fluid. It arrived through the mail in an unmarked package. The user was instructed to add the liquid in the vial to a urine sample while in the privacy of the bathroom before submitting the specimen to the urine collector. Urine Luck oxidized drugs to other compounds, thereby producing a false negative urine drug test result. Jaco tried it out with his at-home drug testing kit and found that it worked for marijuana. By this time, he also began experimenting with heroin. Urine Luck worked on this drug too. Jaco went online and purchased enough of the adulterant to last him for three years of quarterly drug testing.

Back in the lab, Calvin noticed something was now different about #32449's urine. His previous urine samples were odorless and colorless, a reflection of his dilute urine. Now, this sample was not near the threshold value, and had a much deeper yellow color. The creatinine level was also now within normal limits. Calvin thought that maybe #32449 had reformed and was now clean. But then he thought, *I don't buy it. He's doing something else.* On a whim, and totally against the rules, Calvin took a solution of THC and added it to one of #32449's samples that previously tested negative. To his astonishment, the repeated test remained negative, even though the added THC should have produced a positive result.

He is definitely doing something again, Calvin thought. *In order to solve this problem, I have to think like a drug user trying to hide my addiction. What would I do if he were me?* Calvin knew that subjects who are drug tested urinate in the privacy of a bathroom without a witness. Maybe #32499 was adding some chemical to invalidate his test. So he went on Google and typed in "adulteration and urine drug testing." There was a hit for Urine Luck. After reading about how this adulterant worked, Calvin came straight to my office. "Do we have permission to test suspicious urine samples for the presence of adulterants such as this?" he asked, showing me the Internet article. I emphatically replied, "We can't do that today. Taking that sort of action would be viewed as a witch hunt. But I'm part of a group of toxicologists who are trying to get the regulations changed so that we *can* do this type of testing. For now, though, we have to be careful that we don't single anyone out." With that Calvin bit his tongue and went back to his office.

About two years later, fervor about adulteration

practices did lead to changes in the federal drug testing policy. Labs were mandated to check for evidence of adulterants. The new law required testing of all urine samples, not just the suspicious ones. A positive adulterant result was worse for the participant than a positive drug test, because it amounted to fraud. The lab developed tests for adulterants, including Urine Luck.

Calvin couldn't wait until #32449's urine showed up in the lab again. Meanwhile, Jaco had gotten wind of these rule changes. He knew he had to stop using Urine Luck. "Now what am I going to do?" he asked his roommate. The stakes were higher. He'd stopped using marijuana and instead he was using heroin regularly now. Like most addicts, he had to have a hit almost daily and could not quit. He had also become the driver for the elementary school children. Unbeknownst to Calvin, his own daughter, Jenny, was one of Jaco's daily passengers.

Two months after the new drug testing regulation was in force, the results of #32449's urine appeared on Calvin's desk. It was positive for morphine, the heroin metabolite.

"We finally got him," Calvin said to me that day. "Now maybe he can be prosecuted accordingly."

I replied, "This is his first offense. He'll have an opportunity to defend himself. This is not over yet."

Jaco met with a medical review officer, or MRO. He explained that he'd had a clean toxicology record for ten years, and that this was all a big mistake. Jaco had seen a

Seinfeld episode and remembered that Elaine had a positive urine result due to poppy seed ingestion, which contains morphine. He remarked in an innocent tone to the MRO, "I ate a poppy seed bagel yesterday. Could that have had any effect?"

The MRO responded, "Yes, poppy seeds are well known to contain morphine. I'm going to recommend that the bus company put you on probation. From now on you'll have to submit to monthly drug tests and they'll be randomly scheduled. We will also arrange to have someone witness you urinating into a cup. You better clean up your act buddy, real fast."

Hearing the outcome of the MRO's hearing on #32449 and that he was only on probation, Calvin was livid. He became obsessed with trying to prove that #32449 was a drug addict. After a few days of research, he came across an article in a toxicology journal by researchers at the University of Connecticut. The investigators showed that testing urine for the presence of thebaine could be used to confirm poppy seed ingestion. Thebaine is not present in street heroin as it is not derived from the poppy plant. Excited, Calvin showed me the article and asked if the lab could test #32449's urine for thebaine.

"No Calvin," I replied. "You're getting too personally involved in this one case. If you don't drop this, you may face disciplinary action." But Calvin disobeyed. He did set up a test for thebaine and examined #32449's urine without my knowledge or permission. As he'd suspected, the result was negative, indicating that #32449 was lying about his positive test result.

I knew it, damn it, he said to himself. *He is a drug user.*

The next week, Jaco went to work driving the school bus. He had just taken a hit of heroin. It was a rainy day, and his vision was impaired. It didn't help that he was also in an opiate haze. He swerved across the center line and hit a woman and a child in their car head on. The children on the bus were thrown about. There were no seat belts. There were loud screams followed by crying. Miraculously, neither he nor any of the children on the bus were seriously hurt. The driver and passenger of the car, however, both died at the scene, their car crushed by the oncoming speeding bus.

Calvin heard the news on the radio and was horrified. The bus was carrying kids from Jenny's school. A chill ran down his spine. He frantically ran to his office to grab his cell phone to call home. Then he remembered that his wife had taken Jenny to the dentist and that Jenny was going to miss school. She was not on that bus. A crowd in the lab gathered in the break room where the news was being reported on local television. The station interrupted the regularly scheduled daytime soaps. A few minutes later, Calvin's cell phone, which was still in his hands, unexpectedly rang. It was from the police.

*

Testing for adulterants by forensic laboratories continues to evolve and improve in order to catch cheaters of the drug-testing system.

Unfortunately, "garage" chemists also evolve by developing new adulterating agents that are designed to mask positive urine drug test results. Moreover, adulteration testing countermeasures add to the cost of testing the drugs themselves.

I believe there is a good deal of hypocrisy surrounding the federal workplace drug testing laws in the U.S. today. On one hand, drug use while working has its penalties. On the other, it is legal in many states for manufacturers to produce products purposely designed to allow someone to pass a drug test. The scope of testing is also incomplete. For example, the mandated testing for phencyclidine, or Angel Dust, makes little sense when the prevalence of this drug is so low. Meanwhile, the abuse of many other drugs, such as oxycodone, goes on unabated. I realize that testing for a wide panel of drugs is impractical and costly. But improvements in testing policy must be made.

Accident Aftermath

****

Calvin was informed that his wife and family were in a terrible traffic accident. Their car was hit head on by a school bus. The driver and passenger, both belted in the car, died at the scene. In the damaged car, police officers found a purse and wallet belonging to Calvin's wife and identified her from the driver's license. Calvin's business card was also there with his work telephone number. The officer calmly told Calvin that their bodies were being taken to the medical examiner's office. He was then instructed to come to the ME's office within a few hours and identify his wife and child. The morgue attendants needed to clean up the bodies before Calving could see them.

Calvin came into my office and said he had to leave immediately. I did not know at the time but could sense that something terrible had happened. I went into the lab and assigned someone else to take over Calvin's duties. When I heard about a traffic accident with a bus from his coworkers, I suspected the worst.

Police officers arrived at the accident scene within a few minutes after the accident occurred. A witness who heard the screeching noise and loud crash dialed 9-1-1.

When the police and medics arrived, they could see that Jaco was behaving erratically. Officers were trained to look for signs of physiological impairment and intoxication. Field sobriety tests were conducted. While standing, Jaco was instructed by an officer to lift one leg 6 inches above the ground and count out loud by thousands for 30 seconds. Jaco was unable to maintain his balance and he put his foot down after only 15 seconds. In the police report, the officer wrote, "Failed one leg standing test." With both feet on the ground, the policeman asked Jaco to focus on a pencil he held out in front of Jaco's eyes. The police officer slowly moved the pencil from side to side. He noticed that Jaco had difficulty tracking the moving pencil. Jaco's eyes jerked when the pencil moved 25 degrees from center. The officer wrote, "Failed the horizontal gaze nystagmus test." Based on these results, Jaco was put into the squad car and taken to the police station. There, a breathalyzer test was conducted. Jaco blew into the device which registered a 0.15%. This was nearly twice the legal limit for allowable alcohol consumption while operating a motor vehicle. The officers completed a report indicating that Jaco was legally drunk while operating the bus that day. They collected and blood and urine on Jaco and the samples were sent to the crime laboratory for analysis. He was read his rights and put into jail for the evening. Jaco did not have money to hire an attorney. A public defender was appointed to his case. A $100,000 bail was posted by his union and Jaco was released. A few days later, the results of the urine drug test were completed. Jaco's urine tested positive for 6-acetylmorpine and morphine. The drug testing laboratory indicated that these were heroin metabolites.

Based on these forensic findings, Jaco was charged with driving while intoxicated for both alcohol and drugs, negligence, and involuntary manslaughter. His crime did not qualify as voluntary manslaughter because the act did not occur when he was provoked. The district attorney wanted to convict him of "criminally negligent" involuntary manslaughter because he was committing a reckless crime at the time of the accident. A key discussion between the DA and the defendant's lawyer was whether or not the defendant was aware of the risk. Jaco admitted that he abused drugs for many years and had a very clean driving record. Therefore he did not have a consciousness of risk.

"It was rainy that day and the roads were slick," the defending's attorney said. "In examining police records, I found several other accidents that occurred in the city."

"But none of them were due to heroin use and none resulted in the death of a woman and her young child," the DA argued.

The defense attorney argued that his client committed the "unlawful act" of manslaughter. "This was *malum prohibitum* and not *malum in se*" he said to the judge in his private chambers.   The judge and DA knew the distinction, where in *Malum in se* the conduct is bad itself while *malum prohibitum*, the lesser of the two offenses, the conduct is bad because it is prohibited by law.

"My client did not foresee that his actions would be the direct cause of the accident. He was a competent driver and not any more negligent than usual. The major contributory factor was bad weather," the defense attorney concluded.

In the end, Jaco was convicted by a jury of his peers of the unlawful act of manslaughter for the death of Calvin's wife and daughter. He was given a 10-year sentence with probation after 7 years. This was a lesser sentence than what he would have received with negligent manslaughter.

Upon hearing this verdict, Calvin's co-workers at the lab were outraged. I, having testified in court many times, couldn't believe the outcome either.

"That creep should be locked up for the rest of his life," one of my techs said.

"What is the point of drug testing if someone can get off with this sentence," said another. I had no comment and left the break room.

*

Calvin was numbed by the sudden death of his entire family. The funeral was held that weekend. Calvin's parents and friends were in attendance. Some of the people from my lab were there. Many of his co-workers from the lab came. During the service, I sat at the back of the funeral home and paid my respects. I told Calvin to take off as much time as needed. He didn't respond. He had a blank stare on his face. The world that he knew had crumbled overnight. Little did I know then how much things would change?

A few days after the funeral, his family left town. Calvin was left alone in the home he and his wife built for themselves. The newspapers from the last few days were still in his driveway wrapped in plastic. He went outside to retrieve and discard them. But then he decided that while it was extremely painful for him, he wanted to see what the reporters said about the accident. He found the paper from the day after the accident in the metro section. There he read that the bus driver was being held for questioning by the police. Calvin then looked at each of the following days for further news.

The paper from four days after the accident read, "Lab tests showed that the Jaco Jamison was under the influence of drugs and alcohol at the time of the accident that killed a child and her mother. Mr. Jamison's employment as a bus driver for the Sunrise School District has been suspended pending a trial." From his work, Calvin knew that all school bus drivers underwent regular urine drug testing. He then realized that his laboratory does the testing for the Sunrise District. *How could this driver be allowed to work if he abuses drugs?* Calvin thought to himself. *Drug testing is conducted to prevent hiring and using intoxicating drivers. So if he is on drugs, how could he be allowed to....* Then a chill through ran down his spine. *Maybe Jaco is Mr. #32449!* he thought. *Maybe he is the one who killed my family!*

Calvin was now determined at all costs to find out if Jaco was this donor of adulterated urine. He knew that all donors signed the first page of the original chain of custody documents each time they donate urine. The signature is not carried over to the subsequent copies, including the page that accompanies the sample to the laboratory. There was no way to find out who #32449 was from the toxicology lab's document. But Jaco knew the location of the urine collection station. Records identifying the donor would be locked in their files. So the next night, Calvin drove to the urine collection station after their closure. Calvin knew there were no watch guards on duty and no alarms in the building. Most people didn't know what goes on in this building. Calvin broke in through the office window and started looking through the files for the information he wanted. The files were listed numerically according to donor number. He found the drawer containing donors #32000 through #32500. With a few minutes, he found the file marked #32449 toward the back of the drawer. He was now sweating profusely. His heart started racing. His hand was shaking as he held the flashlight. Scanning down the form to the signature line, he found what he was looking for.

Calvin whispered out loud. "Donor #32449 is Jaco Jamison! This is the same man who murdered my family." Then Calvin thought he heard a noise from outside. He found what he was looking for so he quickly replaced the file into its rightful position, closed the file drawer and seeing no one, he left the building.

When he arrived home, Calvin starting thinking about this Jaco person. *The name sounds familiar*, he thought. Calvin saw that the newspaper reported that Jaco was 26 years old. *How do I know this name?* On a hunch, Calvin pulled out his old high school yearbook he bought when he was a freshman. Sure enough, Jaco Jamison went to the same high school and was a senior that year. Looking more closely at the picture and thinking back to his freshman year, jogged his memory. *He's the kid that pushed me in the bathroom! He was a creep even back then. I hope he gets life imprisonment for what he did to my family.*

The first thing in the morning of the next day, Calvin came back to the laboratory, barged into my office and slammed the door. The window of my office shook and nearly shattered under the concussion. I had never seen Calvin so enraged. He was always calm and quiet before.

"I know that donor #32449 was the bus driver who killed my family," he shouted.

"Calvin, calm down. What are you talking about?" I responded.

"He is the donor of that urine sample that I found adulterated. Mr. 32449 killed my family," Calvin reiterated.

"How could you know that? This is confidential information. How did you get this information? You could be held libel...."

"Never mind how I know," Calvin interrupted. I could see he didn't care about any consequences to this breach of confidentiality. I found out and it's him. It's all your fault. I blame YOU for the death of my family."

I was flabbergasted at hearing this rant. *How am I involved?* I asked myself. *What is he saying?*

"We knew this man was a menace to the public. You knew it too, and yet you did NOTHING to get him off the street." Calvin was shouting and crying at the same time. I had never seen this behavior from my former student and employee. "I wanted to report his positive drug test results and urine adulteration practices to the bus company, but you did not allow it. Now my wife and daughter are dead. I hope you go to hell for this!"

I felt about as small as a man could feel. I knew that he was right. We didn't report the result that could have led to Jaco's dismissal as a driver. As he was shouting, I thought of my own family. How devastated I would be if anything happened to them. But I also knew that if we had inappropriately reported this result, my laboratory could be sued, our work suspended, or the lab could have been forced to close. I myself could face criminal charges regarding breech of privacy. None of this knowledge made me feel any better. There was nothing I could say to Calvin to ease his pain. I arose from my desk and tried to reach for him, but he shoved me back.

"Stay away. I never want to see you again," he shouted. He then yelled some more obscenities at me and stomped out of the room. I didn't try to stop him as he left. Several of the lab workers were watching this drama take place. I could sense that many felt I was at fault. I shut the door, turned off the light in my office and sat at my desk in the dark with my head in my hands. *Maybe there could have been something I should have done,* I thought to myself. After

30 minutes, I got up and left the building. My staff was glaring at me as I left. I looked down the entire time and did not make any eye contact. I took sick days off for the remainder of that week.

Over the next few days, I was thinking about quitting my job as the toxicology lab director. I took a few more days off, but by the following week, I returned to the lab to resume my duties. Nobody ever brought up Calvin's case or wanted to discuss the death of his family after the funeral. About two weeks later, I received a letter from Calvin's attorney stating that effective immediately, his client was resigning his post in my laboratory. The attorney left instructions as to where his final paycheck was to be sent. I passed the letter on to our human resources office. The next day, that office posted a job opening to fill Calvin's position that was now vacant. I was not surprised that Calvin resigned. I hoped he could find peace with himself.

*

Calvin left town and flew to Barbados. He didn't tell anyone where he was going or when or if he would return. Calvin was not an alcoholic and never drank heavily before. But now he needed something to forget about his troubles. He developed a taste for tequila and drank every night while he was away. He passed out in his room and slept for 14-18 hours. He would not wake up until late in the afternoon the following day. Calvin would eat something, but then start drinking heavily again. After a week of this behavior, he realized he had to stop and resume his life. But he had quit his job at my lab and he didn't know what to do or where to go. He couldn't live in the house that he and his wife had built. The memories were too painful. He planned to put his house on the market when he returned and move to a new city to start over. He needed a job as he was just 33 years old. But what was he going to do? He felt the clinical toxicology field let him down and he no longer valued it as a profession. Yet this was all that he knew. Calvin was sitting in the bar when someone approached him. The man sat down next to him and started a casual conversation. This chance meeting was going to change everything.

In order to make their plan work for the company, they needed a biochemist. Someone who was smart and willing to work on products that were a little outside the norm. Since Calvin used to work for me, he remembered what happened to one of the graduate students that used to work in my department. Cao Pham was arrested for keeping anthrax in his lab shortly after the 9-1-1 attack. He left graduate school after his second girlfriend died a tragic death. From his old school, Calvin obtained Cao's contact information and asked if he was interested in joining Test-Me Inc. Cao had done some protein synthesis while in grad school and accepted the job.

*

A patient's medical information is protected by the Health Insurance Portability and Accountability Act (HIPAA) of 1996. There are stiff penalties and criminal charges that can be filed for individuals violating an individual's private information. Although there are different interpretations that have been rendered, workplace urine drug testing is not considered medical information. Donors for drug testing are not patients and the testing is not conducted for diagnostic or medical purposes. Therefore most states have the prevailing view that drug test results are not PHI (protected health information) and HIPAA regulations do not apply. Nevertheless, there are other privacy laws that govern the release of workplace drug testing information and Calvin violated these laws. As someone who was made aware of this violation, I was negligent in not reporting this breach in confidentiality. Given what Calvin went through, I was reluctant to report his indiscretion. It was also unclear who I would report him to? He was no longer my employee and the bus company had already discharged Jaco from his job and he was currently serving a prison sentence.

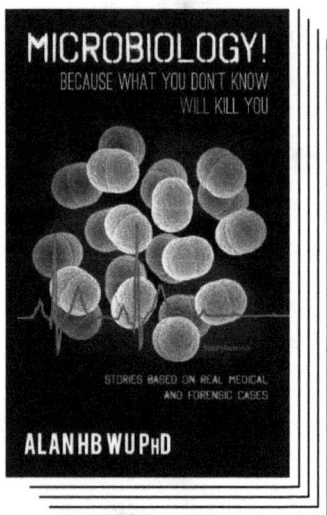

MICROBIOLOGY!
BECAUSE WHAT YOU DON'T KNOW
WILL KILL YOU

STORIES BASED ON REAL MEDICAL
AND FORENSIC CASES

ALAN HB WU PhD

Mysophobia

****

She started out as a comedian. She was a regular at the *Standup*, a comedy night club in Manhattan Beach and performed to a small audience of about 50 people on Friday nights along with other Hollywood wannabes. Jason Allen was also a regular at the club and appeared on Saturday nights. He was not available during the week, as he was busy in Culver City filming of *After Hours Show with Jason Allen*. The club's manager, Jason's long-time friend, told him about Connie and showed Jason some video footage of her act. She joked that she was single because she was afraid of direct physical contact with humans.

"I never shake hands with anyone who I meet for the

first time," she said during one of her gigs. "Especially men. Men are disgusting. I've seen how my older brothers behave. They gorge themselves with spicy foods and then take turns trying to out burp and out fart each other. My brother would extend his hand, and when you shook it, there would be this prolonged audible leakage of noxious vapor. It takes talent to regulate your anal sphincter like a high-pressure methane gas regulator. Then when it was time to go to the bathroom, they would sit there for 15 minutes or more, reading car racing magazines the whole while. So naturally when I meet strange men for the first time, I can only think back to when I was a kid. *'Where has THAT hand been?'* I would ask myself." This always got a laugh and sort of became her trademark line. It was these childhood memories that caused Connie to have mysophobia, a fear of germs. Jason was amused but bathroom humor was never his style. Fortunately, Connie commented on other differences between men and women and she had a nice comedic delivery.

At Jason's request, the club manager invited Connie to be an opening act for Jason during one of his Saturday *Standup* shows. She got lots of laughs from the crowd and it got them in a good mood for Jason's monologue. At the end of the night, Connie was summoned to meet Jason in his dressing room. When he extended his hand, Connie raised both her hands up, palms out, and did not grab Jason's hand to shake it.

"So this is real? You really are a germaphobe?" he asked her.

"Yeah, I have been all my life. But this interferes with my social life," she told him.

Her attitude towards physical contact was just the opposite of Jason's. At the beginning of his shows, he shook hands and "high fived" dozens of the people from the studio audience who came to see him. This rapport served him well during his entire *After Hours Show* run of 15 years. After a few minutes of talk in his dressing room, Jason told her that he was going to give her a guest spot on television. Through his show, Jason had launched the careers of many comedians, just like Johnny Carson did decades before him. Naturally, Connie was thrilled. She jumped up and was about to hug him, but then composed herself. *Where has HE been?* was her germaphobic thought. She gave him her contact information and Jason left the nightclub and his driver took him home.

Connie appeared on Jason's show a few months later. The television studio audience loved her. Instead of a music number that night, Connie's bit was the closing act of the show. There wasn't time for her to be an actual guest and sit with Jason while on the air. Since she lived in the Los Angeles area, the *After Hours Show* producers would sometimes call her to substitute for a guest who cancelled at the last minute and she became somewhat of a regular guest host. While she was never the head-lining guest, she did get to sit in the guest chair to the left of Jason and the audience got to know her a little better. Connie had an engaging personality and Jason never had to worry about filling up time with her like he sometimes had to do with some of the celebrities that were booked. He genuinely liked her and was happy to have her on the show from time to time.

The studios took notice of how comfortable she was in front of a camera. A few years later a producer asked her to audition to be a host of a new daytime game show called *Family Fights*. She made the shortlist of candidates, all but her were men. She was told that it was a show where families compete against other families with a series of questions and perform physical tasks. During the introduction, Connie was asked to introduce the families and question them about their lives. Connie was brilliant during a practice run of the show and she was pegged to be the new show's host. The show was mildly popular on the game show network, but never made it to any of the major networks or on prime time. It was only after she was offered the job that she told them that she had mysophobia. The producers agreed that the host did not have any physical contact with contestants, and that the studio would keep multiple containers of hand sanitizers on the set.

*

Connie's only outlet from work was playing soccer. She was a goalie on a club team in Pasadena where she lived. She had played throughout high school and was the goalie. This position did not require much physical contact with her sweaty teammates or any of the players which suited her well. She told her teammates from the very beginning that giving "high-fives" was not her thing. They competed against other teams in the area. One of the games was played on artificial turf. She had never played on such a surface before and was amazed at how fast the ball moved. During one play, she dove to her left to successfully block a shot. Her team won the game that day, but when she returned home, she noticed that her right knee had a nasty scrape as the result of the shot she saved. She put antiseptic ointment on it, covered the wound with a bandage and didn't think anything further about it.

Within a few days, however, the wound on her knee did not heal and instead became infected. She put on more neosporin. Soon, other lesions began to appear on other parts of her body including her face. At first, she was able to cover up the outbreak with makeup. But when it did not get better, the show's producers were forced to put her show on temporary hiatus. They told her to see a doctor.

Connie arrived at the General on a Thursday. She was immediately placed into the ICU ward under isolation. Nobody was allowed in her room unless they wore special sterile gowns, gloves, and masks. There was a sink outside her door and everyone exiting the room had to wash their hands.

Sputum and blood samples were sent to the laboratory for cultures. At the time, we did not offer a molecular test for the causative agent. So it took several days before the identity of the bacterial agent could be made. In the meantime, Connie was treated with a wide spectrum antibiotic. Eventually, she was diagnosed with *Staphylococcus aureus.* It was later determined that this particular strain of bacteria was resistant to beta lactam-type antibiotics such as penicillin and methicillin. It was termed MRSA, or methicillin-resistant *Staph aureus.*

*

As part of our training program to laboratory medical technology students and postdoctoral fellows, we go on lab medicine "rounds" whereby we regularly visit patient wards and discuss relevant clinical laboratory tests results. Most clinical laboratorians spend their entire day in the lab and never see how their results are actually being used to make medical decisions. These sessions are hosted by our pathology residents who review case histories and provide a summary of clinical laboratory test findings to the group. On one day in particular, the resident selected Connie's case. When I found out that we were discussing a public figure, I warned my staff that disclosure of a patient's medical information to anyone who is not part of the patient's healthcare team was prohibited and can result in significant fines and criminal charges to those who violate patient privacy. We were justified in attending because we provide laboratory results that are part of patient care. With this preface, my resident proceeded cautiously to present her case. We did not gown up and enter her isolated room. As such, she could not hear what was being said and was asleep in her bed. But through the observation window, we could clearly see extensive pus-filled lesions throughout her face, arms, and legs. These parts of her skin were not covered because blankets would have caused skin irritation. To me, her appearance was dramatically different from what she looked like on television. She was hardly recognizable.

The resident described the laboratory procedure that was conducted in order to diagnose this infection. "Under the microscope, Staphylococcus, as the name implies, are round, globe-shaped organisms that turn blue with the application of the Gram stain. We then grew colonies from a blood culture sample using an appropriate media. Biochemical tests from colonies taken from the culture are performed to determine that this is *Staphlycoccus aureus* and not some other coccal bacteria."

"How did she contract this?" one of my students asked.

My laboratory medicine resident responded, "From the medical record, it appears to have started from an abrasion suffered playing soccer on a field that contained an artificial turf. There have been many cases of MRSA infection amongst athletes, although in most cases, it was infections spread in the locker room by sharing towels or not sanitizing whirlpools."

While we were standing there, several other doctors were leaving her room and removing their personal protective equipment. Each of them thoroughly washed their hands. While they were doing that, I started singing the "*Happy Birthday*" song quietly, but loud enough so that my students could hear me but the doctors near the sink couldn't. One of the newer students, Fay, looked at me and

I could tell that she thought I was off my rocker. But most of the other students knew what I was doing. I explained to Fay that the proper duration for hand washing is the same amount of time needed to sing this song.

"I tell all my students to do this which serves as a reminder to not short cut this important infection control step," I told her.

While my resident continued on with his discussion, Fay was watching the next doctor who went to wash his hands. I could tell that she was singing this song in her mind, and each of the doctors had cleansed themselves properly. I didn't mind that I had distracted some of my students away from the discussion at hand. *This lesson for Fay was far more important than the details of Connie's case*, I thought to myself.

"They all did it long enough. It works!" she said to me off to the side.

Learning from my resident that Connie suffered from mysophobia, I said to Fay, "Our patient would have approved of the hand washing practices performed by her doctors."

*

Connie had a severe case of MRSA and spent the next month in the hospital. Her lifestyle of repeated hand washing made her susceptible to an infection because it removed her resident skin flora, making it easier for the opportunistic MRSA strain to invade. Connie suffered scars from the infection on her body and face. Her show was cancelled. Because of her altered appearance, she was not given any new opportunities in Hollywood. This is a tough town that cherishes beauty. While Connie was never gorgeous, the producers did not want anyone on camera with a liability in their appearance.

An infectious disease specialist told Connie that her excessive hand sanitation practices contributed to her contracting a MRSA infection. She was lucky that her infection did not affect her organs like her heart. Connie was told to see a psychiatrist to treat her affliction. Wanting to be more normal, she complied. She was diagnosed with "blood-infection-injury phobia" and obsessive-compulsive disorder. She was treated by a technique known as "cognitive behavior therapy." A female therapist created exercises to help her over her affliction. The therapist would thoroughly wash her hands in front of Connie to show that she was clean. Then she told Connie to massage the therapist's hands including the cracks between all of her fingers on both hands. Connie cognitively knew there were no germs, but she had never touched someone's hands in this way before. In later sessions, the exercise would be repeated except the therapist would wash her hands out of Connie's direct view. Later still, a man came and performed the exercise. Eventually, there was no hand washing in her presence, and she was told to trust them.

These counseling sessions were effective and her mysophobia abated considerably. Connie left the Los Angeles area and moved to Texas where she got married and became a mom shortly thereafter. Later she became a soccer coach when her children grew older. None of her children suffered from a fear of germs.

*

A few weeks after we attended rounds on Connie, I was summoned to appear in front of one of our privacy officers. These individuals regularly monitor who has access to private medical records and it was noticed that one of my residents had electronically accessed her file. Since Connie was a celebrity she was put on a special list, and I had to justify why it was necessary. I told them that Connie's MRSA infection was unusual in terms of how severe it was and how she contracted it. The privacy officer knew that most hospital cases were spread from contact with healthcare workers. "This was not the case here, but we used this as an example of the importance sanitation to avoid hospital-acquired infections." As we are a university hospital, this was an acceptable justification for our file review. But then I received the standard privacy warning regarding future encounters. *Celebrities are no different from other patients,* I thought to myself as I was leaving his office.

*

Staphylococcus aureus *is a common gram-positive bacterium that is found in the skin and the anterior nares of the nose. It is part of resident flora and produces no harm. For some individuals, however, a Staph infection can cause skin infections manifested by pimples, boils, and abscesses. These bacteria exert their pathologic damage by releasing chemicals that are toxic to human cells.*

Through bacterial resistance, nature has created a

pathway that enables some of the bacteria to escape destruction by man-made drugs. Over the years, these microorganisms have mutated in such a way that penicillin-like drugs are no longer effective. Infections by methicillin-resistant Staphylococcus aureus can cause significant illnesses if not treated early and effectively. Fortunately, there are next-generation antibiotics that are effective against MRSA. Many states including California require reporting of hospital-acquired MRSA, estimated to be about 85% of all cases, with appropriate isolation of patients who are colonized.

Connie was not the only game show host who was afraid of direct human contact. Deal or No Deal's Howie Mandel's germaphobic aversion is well chronicled in his autobiography, Here's the Deal: Don't Touch Me. There he described a chronic obsessive disorder that caused him to wash his hands repeatedly and use hand sanitizers when a sink was not readily available. As a child, he never re-tied his shoelaces when they came undone because of the laces' exposure to the ground. In hotels, he would carry an ultraviolet light in an attempt to eliminate bacteria. He admits that his removal of germs on his body has probably made him more prone to infections than normal. This may have occurred with Connie as well.

Transmission of MRSA through exposure from artificial turf has been described previously. Materials used to produce these playing surfaces are known to retain the viability of bacteria, which promotes infection of unsuspecting athletes. Several members of the Tampa Bay Buccaneers professional football team have been infected with MRSA, thought to have occurred through open wounds created by the abrasive surface of fake grass. Sanitizing artificial turf is not yet regularly performed. Fortunately, these fields are slowly being replaced by natural turf because they are softer and are associated with fewer injuries.

It was ironic that Connie was always fearful of an infection from human contact. Despite her precautions, she unknowingly became infected by another female goalie who was on the field before her, and left some of her body fluids on the playing field.

The Hand Sanitizer

Connie's life in Texas was great for the first 20 years of her marriage to Harold. They had one child together. Unfortunately, it all began to unravel once her children became young adults and left home. Her daughter, Casey, wanted to follow her mother's footsteps and moved to Los Angeles to become a television personality. Harold was busy with his business travels leaving Connie alone at home. Harold and Connie started to drift apart. They mutually agreed to separate and ultimately were divorced. She received an excellent settlement because Texas is one of nine states in the U.S. that has community property jurisdiction. She relocated to the Northern California Bay Area because of the better weather in the summer of 2017.

With her settlement, and the sale of their family home in Texas, Connie bought a small home in the East Bay. Her mysophobia, which was somewhat controlled while she was married and raising Casey, started to re-surface. She also started suffering from oniomania, compulsive buying disorder. She went to many different stores on a daily basis to purchase items she thought she needed. Soon, her garage was filled with books, clothing, lamps, and furniture. She also started to stockpile household items in her basement, including canned goods, bags of potato chips and other junk food items, bottled water and other beverages, and breakfast cereal boxes. She bought several deep freezers and loaded them with meats and vegetables. She loaded up the bathroom with paper goods. Connie had cases of sanitary napkins even though she was postmenopausal and hadn't had a period in 5 years. Her daily appearance also began to suffer. Her clothing was in disarray and her hair was dirty and un-kept. The toilet paper was stacked on three walls from the floor to the ceiling. She thought to herself, *the safest place to be during a hurricane or earthquake is the bathroom. Now I am doubly protected.* She covered up her bathroom mirrors. *I know what I look like, I don't need to be reminded,* she said to herself as her rationale.

Word got around Hollywood that Connie had fallen from grace. Freelance paparazzi found her home address, and waited in vehicles on the street outside her home, and took pictures when she came out to take in her mail. These photos were sold to tabloid newspapers for all to see. Considering that she was once a TV game show host, this came as quite a shock when her old friends saw current pictures of her. Some of them tried to reach out to her to see if they could help, but Connie did not respond to their telephone calls, text messages or emails.

Connie's mysophobia was also part of the spectrum of her obsessive-compulsive disorder. Like before, she began to avoid contact with anyone. She would not shake hands with acquaintances and stayed at least 6 feet apart from any stranger. She wore gloves to handle anything including doorknobs, shopping carts and elevator buttons. When she received mail, she sprayed each piece with disinfectant prior to opening them. Connie's mysophobia went into another gear when she read that coronavirus can live on cardboard for 24 hours, wood for 2 days, and plastics and glass for 4 days.

In the store, she maintained 6 feet of "social distancing" between patrons. This was years before this term entered the nation's everyday vernacular due to the COVID pandemic. All of her store purchases were made with credit-cards, there was never any exchange of bills or coins. She would insist to the clerks that she swipe the card through the machine herself. She would then wipe her card before returning it to a clear plastic bag. Connie would not allow anybody from the store to bag her groceries or help load them into her car. She had sanitizers in her hatchback vehicle to use immediately after loading. Once at home, she would thoroughly wash her hands and disinfected her shopping bags.

Casey tried to get Connie to seek psychiatric care but her mother refused. She maintained a daily routine that did not vary by the day of the week. She read the newspaper each morning and listened to the network news broadcasts on TV in the evening. During the day, she would drive to the store and buy items that she didn't need or really want. When she learned about how she can receive purchased goods through Amazon Prime home delivery, she stopped going to stores and she rarely needed to leave her neighborhood. At this point, she was now a certified recluse.

*

The COVID-19 infection had an effect on everybody on the planet. The effect on Connie was in some respect a validation of her behavior while ultimately being catastrophic. In December of 2019, she followed the daily reports originating from a relatively unknown city of Wuhan, China regarding a new coronavirus. Unlike most Americans at the time, she was fearful that this could eventually affect the rest of the world. She went online and purchased several cases of masks, face shields, gloves, sterile gowns, bleach, and hand sanitizers. Before long, her supply of goods mimicked a mini-Costco.

She called Casey and told her to do the same.

"Mom, what are you doing? There is not going to be a problem. There was a small coronarvirus outbreak back in 2003 and hardly anybody here got infected," Casey said to her mother.

"No, No! It's coming. We have to prepare. WE HAVE TO PREPARE! I will send you some of my supplies. They are going to run out. Yes, there will be a demand for these. You'll see. I'm right. I will send you supplies. Toilet paper! Do you have enough? I will order you some. We have to protect ourselves. I know I am right." Connie was ranting. Casey had seen this behavior before and was fearful that her OCD was going to take over her personality.

In February of 2020, Connie read about the first

cases to appear in America. *Its starting*, she thought. *I need to get more supplies. There will be a mad rush to the grocery store and I might be out of luck.* In reality, she had enough groceries to shelter down for 12 months or more. She went online and ordered more food, water, and disposable supplies. She bought a large-capacity gasoline-powered generator in case the electricity went out. She also purchased 100 tanks of propane and several outdoor barbecues. Of course these units had to be new. She went to hardware stores and purchased hundreds of packs of batteries of all sizes. She already had 25 flashlights, but she went to several stores to buy 50 more. When she started to run out of space, she went to a lumber yard and purchased utility sheds. She wanted to buy a large 10,000 gallon below ground gasoline tank, but nobody would install it in for a private citizen.

*

The pandemic hit a feverish pitch in America in March of 2020, prompting President Donald Trump to shut down un-essential businesses, and ordering the citizens to shelter-in-place. Never before in the history of the U.S. had such an order been placed. Within days, all stores and restaurants were closed. The parks and streets were empty. Buses and trains carried 10% of their normal load. Traffic jams disappeared. All sporting, concerts, and religious ceremonies were postponed or cancelled. The country went into a recession with large segments of the population being laid off their jobs and consumer spending went down to a trickle. The travel and entertainment industry took the biggest hit. The stock market, especially the Dow Jones Index, took unprecedented declines.

News of the spreading coronavirus sent Connie into a deeper mysophobic mode. She stopped going outside entirely. Every day she received dozens of boxes. Once the contents were brought in, she broke down the boxes and stacked them into the corner of her porch. Soon, this area was completely filled with these boxes. Neighbors tried to call and come by to complain, but Connie would not talk to them.

*

The pandemic greatly affected Calvin's business. Sales of his adulteration drugs were down. If this continued, he would have to lay off his staff. He assembled his team via a teleconference call to ask how Test-Me, Inc. could profit from the pandemic. Having been a lab tech working in a hospital, he knew that there would be shortages of personal protective equipment such as masks, gloves, and gowns.

"But we're not a clothing company. We don't have access to the raw materials and machines for production of PPE," Cao said.

But Calvin, who is always on the ball when it comes to making money, had another idea. "We are basically a chemical company. The country will need disinfectants and hand sanitizers. Let's get to work on producing these for sale."

"Typically, these products contain 80% ethanol or 75% isopropyl alcohol. To save money, let's formulate with the latter, rubbing alcohol," Cao suggested. Calvin agreed. We asked the group if they should put fruity aromas to the product in order to make it more attractive. They agreed to add apple, strawberry, and lemon scents to the formulae. In order to save on labor costs, Test-Me, Inc. contracted with a chemical company in Mexico. They got a low dollar quote from one company and were selected to be their supplier. Cao sent them a formula and soon they were producing thousands of gallons of disinfectant which they poured into inexpensive hand pump dispensers. The products were now being sold to their customers. What Calvin and Cao didn't know was that this company had the lowest price because they made a critical substitution with the key ingredient. The company was deceptive as they sent sample product containing the right elements, which therefore passed all of Test-Me's quality control analyses.

*

During the middle of the pandemic, there was a nationwide shortage of PPE and sanitizing solution. While she still had crates full of the product, Connie had the compulsion to purchase more. Connie search through internet sites and came across Test-Me's product. She immediately ordered several thousand bottles to ensure that she would not run out. When the product arrived, she was delighted with the fruity aroma of the sanitizers and began using it daily. Connie put this product on her hands multiple times per hour, and she used up several bottles per day. It took about a week before she became ill from using this tainted hand sanitizer. It first started with a headache. Then it progressed to tingling on her fingers and toes. Then her vision became affected. She did not know what was happening to her body. The very last thing she wanted to do was to go to a hospital and be infected by other patients and healthcare workers who may be infected with COVID-19. A few days later, she started having seizures and became totally blind. That evening, Connie went into a coma and never recovered. It would be days before the rotting smell of her corpse permeated the neighborhood. Her home already smelled of garbage and refuge, so it took a little longer for the neighbors to notice. When the police came in, they found Connie's rotting body on the bathroom floor next to her cathedral of toilet paper.

*

Jacob, my postdoctoral fellow was doing a rotation at the medical examiner's office to train using their forensic toxicology methods, when Connie's body arrived. Without a history of illness just prior to her death, a complete toxicology screen was conducted for prescription and recreational drugs, heavy metals, and volatile alcohols. It was good experience for Jacob as we don't offer heavy metal testing or toxic alcohols. We only routinely measure ethyl alcohol. The ME's office's toxicology laboratory also uses a different method for measuring alcohols. In the hospital, we use an enzymatic assay that is specific for the alcohol found in drinks, while they use a procedure known as "head-space gas chromatography" that tests for the presence of wood alcohol, rubbing alcohol, and acetone in addition to ethanol. Investigators from the medical examiner's office went into Connie's home and found many empty containers of hand sanitizers and they suspected that they would find either ethanol or isopropyl alcohol in her remains. Unused bottles were confiscated for testing as well. Because Connie's body had degraded and partially mummified, samples from the vitreous of her eyes were taken and tested. This body fluid is a preferred site for collection and testing as it is better preserved. To everybody's surprise, the lab found a high concentration of methanol, with only a trace amount of isopropyl alcohol.

The Poison Control Center was contacted and they sent their investigators into Connie's home to determine the source of this toxic form. Among the items they confiscated were near-empty containers of the hand sanitizer bottles that were lying about the house. When the toxicology laboratory tested several representative bottles, high levels of methanol were found in all of them. The Chief Pathologist ruled the cause of Connie's death was accidental due to methanol poisoning. The FDA was alerted to the presence of methanol in Test-Me's product. The product was recalled, and a public warning was issued by the FDA about the dangers of using hand sanitizers containing methanol. Calvin made a statement that his company was not responsible for Connie's death as they did not produce the product. The Mexican company who supplied Calvin had vacated its operation, and the owners could not be located.

Casey and a handful of former Hollywood friends and acquaintances attended Connie's funeral. The morticians did a great job making Connie look like she did when she was on television, decades before. There were pictures of her surrounding the casket showing her on the set of *Family Fights*, when she was the game show's host. The tabloids covered her death with a story and photographs published near the back pages of their rag.

*

Unlike ethanol, which is found in all alcohol beverages, methanol is toxic to humans. Methanol breaks down to formaldehyde which can cause blindness, and formic acid which produces a metabolic disturbance. Methanol is found in some household fluids such as windshield wiper fluid, paint thinners, and various cleaning products. A small amount of methanol can be found in wine. In addition to neurologic problems, individuals with methanol poisoning can also suffer from cardiac effects. Individuals with toxic concentrations of methanol can be treated with ethanol, which retards the rate by which the toxic metabolites form. They can also be given fomepizole, a drug that also retards the rate of methanol metabolism. Connie did not call for medical assistance to enable use of either of these countermeasures.

Excessive use of hand sanitizers can result in absorption of the alcohol through the skin. Levels can exceed the legal driving limit in blood or alcohol of 0.08%. Because methanol is highly toxic, a blood concentration exceeding 0.08% can be fatal if not treated.

Connie did not die of a COVID-19 infection. She could, however, be considered a victim of "collateral damage." Her mysophobic affliction combined with the world health situation were the major factors in her death. Undoubtedly, there have been many other individuals who have died due to the stress of contracting this virus. While it has been well documented that individuals with co-morbidities such as diabetes and hypertension are at greater risk for an infection, psychiatric disease is not recognized as an important factor. It is clear that mysophobics are susceptible to infections having reduced normal microbial flora. Connie did survive a MRSA infection. However, her behavior and unlucky circumstance of a global pandemic led to her demise.

Connie did not suffer for the psychiatric disorder commonly known as "hoarding." This disease is characterized by in an individual's inability to discard items. These people often frequent their neighbor's garbage and retrieve items they deemed to be valuable.

On July 27, 2020, the FDA reiterated a warning that they originally sent in June, about the dangers of using methanol-containing hand sanitizers. The agency felt it necessary because of increasing calls to poison centers from exposed individuals. A "do-not-use list" of dangerous hand sanitizer products was issued by the FDA. Unfortunately, there are other products that have not been reported or labeled as containing methanol that are being sold. To be safe, consumers should only use products from reputable manufacturers.

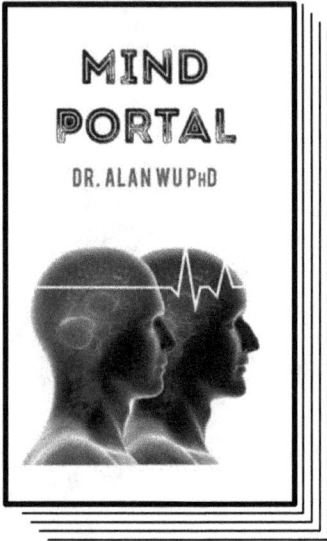

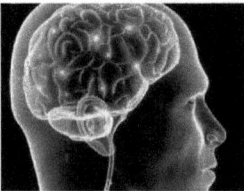

Mind Portal: How it Began

****

They came from Mumbai and settled in Sunnyvale, California. The father was a brilliant software engineer and he worked for one of the pioneering companies in a region that became the Silicon Valley. After a few years, he and his wife had a son. They named him Amit, which in Indian, means "limitless." He would be their only child. Amit was a small boy for his age. In the early 1960s there weren't that many Indian families living on the San Francisco Peninsula. He was shy, and somewhat of an outcast. He had few friends. Many of the other kids in his school lived on farms and orchards that were abundant in the area then. These kids had nothing in common with Amit who had darker skin.

From his early teenage years, Amit Savjani knew that God had given him a unique gift. He could look at someone and not only know what they were thinking but also he could plant thoughts into their mind. He first discovered this ability on the school's courtyard when the school bully, Samuel, was trying to take Amit's lunch money. Samuel had numerous fights with other boys in school. The much larger kid saw Amit from across the courtyard and went over to him with an angry and determined look on his face. Samuel was sporting a thin beard while Amit had not yet begun to shave.

Amit knew he could not avoid Samuel so he braced himself for a face-to-face confrontation. Their eyes locked on each other despite the height difference. There were no words spoken. They just stared at each other for a solid two minutes. All the other kids stopped their conversation and what they were doing to watch this confrontation. There was total silence on the courtyard. Some of the girls were fearful that Amit was going to get hurt but they stood motionless and powerless to say or do anything. Nobody left to get help.

With deep concentration, Amit began sending out his thoughts from his mind to Samuel's. He didn't know why he would try this. Amit was just hoping for a better outcome. *You don't want to do this. This is not right. You are a* good person. *We could be friends. You don't want to do this.* At first, there was nothing. But after another minute passed, Amit could see that it was working. Samuel was getting the non-verbal message. He backed off a step and dropped his head. His facial expression went from aggressive and angry to calm and friendly. His conscience was talking to him. *I don't need to do this. This is not right. I am a good person. We could be friends. I won't do this.* Samuel extended his arm and he and Amit shook hands. Samuel then put his arm around the smaller boy's shoulder.

"Maybe you can help me with my homework," he said to Amit. "I have trouble with just about everything."

"Sure, anytime," Amit remarked with a renewed sense of confidence. Samuel backed away. He thought, *why did I say that to that kid? I was going to pound him into the ground. I don't give a crap about school. What has gotten into me?* He shrugged off these thoughts and left the schoolyard. He went to his car in the school's parking lot for a beer and a smoke.

The kids who were watching this could not believe this transformation. Some of the other boys who were playing basketball and stopped to watch were noticeably disappointed. "Damn, I was looking forward to a good fight," one of them said.

"Naw, it wouldn't have lasted long," another said. "Look at that puny Indian kid. He would have folded into a heap."

"I suppose you're right," the first kid remarked. "But we haven't had a good fight in a long time. What else is there to do here besides gawk at the girls?" The boys went back to their game.

On the other side of the courtyard, a group of girls were also commenting. "Who is that Indian boy? There was something about his look that defused the situation."

One of the more attractive girls commented. "I don't know who this boy is, but I am going to get to know him. He has something special. Unlike that loser Samuel, this kid is going places." A few minutes later, the class bell rang, and recess was over. The students slowly headed back to resume their classes. There was a continuous murmur of what they had witnessed.

Amit wasn't sure what had just happened. He didn't plan on staring down Samuel and he had no reason to believe it would work. But at the critical moment of his confrontation, he had no fear. He knew that he could transmit his thoughts to the bigger, older boy. He went home that night with a confidence that he never had before. He did not tell his mother or father about what happened that day or what he was able to do. He needed to know if he could do it again and learn the limits of his mind.

*

Amit graduated from high school and was admitted to college. He majored in biochemistry and excelled in his classes. He also minored in world history. It was an unusual mix. Amit realized that his future vocation was likely science, but he felt a connection with individuals who made major accomplishments during their lifetimes.

In his sophomore year, Amit was enrolled in an organic chemistry class. During the laboratory portion of the course, he was paired with Angie as a lab mate. Together they worked on the chemistry experiments assigned by the professor. Angie was very attractive and smart. Amit thought that she would never be interested in him romantically. Over the next few weeks, they became friends and they would often meet to have coffee. One day, Amit asked Angie about her weekend plans, hoping that she was free so he could ask her out.

"I got fixed up with a guy named Carl." Angie lived in a sorority that was friendly with one of the fraternities on campus. *I wish that was me,* Amit thought.

"We're going out hiking by the dish." There is a park with a radio telescope near the campus where students go to exercise and relax. Amit looked into Angie's eyes and after a brief moment, he saw a vision that noticeably startled him. Angie saw that Amit's expression had dramatically changed.

"What?" Angie asked. "Why are you looking at me like that?"

"I'm sorry, I didn't mean to stare. It's just that, that... Oh, it's nothing. I hope you have a good time," Amit said.

Angie sensed that Amit was attracted to her. But she didn't want to encourage him, so she said nothing further. *I've never seen him like this. He's acting weird,* she thought. After a few minutes, she said she had to go to class, and she departed without looking back.

Amit remained in the coffee shop and was in great distress. He had seen in Angie's eyes that she was going to be raped by her date in the park that weekend. But he wasn't sure if it was real, so he hadn't said anything to her. He didn't know what to do. *Should I warn her? Should I call the campus police? What real evidence do I have? He'll deny his intentions and I will look foolish. Should I follow her on her date? If she saw me following her, she would really think I am a weirdo.* In the end, Amit sat in his dorm room on that early Saturday evening and did nothing hoping that his vision was wrong. But somehow, he knew he was right.

Unfortunately, Angie during their date was assaulted by Carl when they were in a secluded part of the park. "Stop! What do you think you're doing?" she pleaded with him as he groped her.

"I know you want this bitch. Shut up and enjoy it," Carl said.

She saw rage in Carl's eyes. Fearful that she would be harmed, Angie did not resist any further. After it was over, Angie left the park alone and ran to her dorm room. The following day, she called her parents who came and took her home. They called the police and charges were filed against Carl. Angie was so upset that she dropped out of school. Carl was convicted of rape and was given a prison sentence. Angie did not return to school. Amit never saw Angie again.

When Amit heard the news, he was crushed that he had done nothing to prevent the attack on Angie. Over and over for the next few weeks, he agonized about the options he could have taken to prevent this attack. He let down his classmate and felt cowardly and depressed. He questioned his maker. *Why was I given this ability? What am I supposed to do with this? What good is it? I don't want this!* While his grades suffered temporarily, nobody knew the torment he was facing. He wanted to call Angie at her home to tell her what he had sensed in that coffee shop but decided against it. She would not believe him and it would serve no purpose.

For the remainder of the semester, Amit got no more visions and he immersed himself into his classes. The chemistry professor assigned another individual to be his lab partner during the course, but it wasn't the same as being with Angie. This made him realize that he loved Angie and regretted that he had never told her of his feelings. Two years later, Amit received his undergraduate degree and enrolled in graduate school majoring in clinical laboratory science. He was hoping to become a professor at a major university medical center.

During his third year of grad school, another event occurred that would change his view of reality. He read in the newspaper that Carl had served his time in prison for his attack on Angie and was released on parole. While in prison, Carl had been trained as an auto mechanic and when he was released, the prison arranged a job for him at a local garage. Somehow, Amit knew the garage where Carl was employed. A few months later, Amit brought his old car into that garage. Carl had never met Amit and didn't know about his connection with Angie. Amit asked for an oil change, tune up and tire rotation, but his real objective was to study Carl. While in the waiting room, Amit focused his attention on the mechanic. Amit's eyes followed Carl's every move. After a while, Amit sensed that Carl had rehabilitated and that he was sorry for his rape of Angie. Amit was able to get Carl to think back about his attack on Angie. *That is not who I am now.* Carl thought. *If I could start college again, my attitude and behavior would be very different.* Amit sat back in the waiting room and wished that he too could go back and start college again. He missed Angie and wished she was in his life in some manner or another. Lost in these thoughts, he was startled when Carl came back to the waiting room to speak with him.

"I noticed when changing your tires that your brake pads are worn to a dangerous level," Carl said. "You should get them fixed."

"Can you do that now?" Amit asked.

"It is 5 o'clock and we're closing soon. But if you bring the car back tomorrow, I will do it first thing in the morning," Carl said.

"Ok, I'll be back." This will give me a chance to study Carl some more, Amit thought. Throughout that evening, Amit kept playing the "what if" game again in his mind. *How would things be different if I could have prevented that attack? If I had seen Carl before the date, maybe I could have changed his intention with my thoughts such as I had done with Samuel that bully from junior high school.* Thinking that he had lost his e happiness, Amit went to sleep in his apartment.

The next morning, he arose and drove to Carl's garage. When he arrived, Carl was nowhere to be seen and another mechanic came to greet him.

"What can I do for you today, sir?" he asked.

"I have an appointment with Carl to have my brake pads replaced," Amit said.

There was a hesitation. "You must be in the wrong place, man. I am the owner of this garage and there is no one by the name of Carl here."

"What? He was working on my car yesterday. I sat right there waiting," Amit pointed to a chair in the waiting room. "I was reading THIS magazine," as Amit pointed to an issue of *Newsweek*.

"Look buddy, I was here all day yesterday and you weren't here. I don't have time to play games. I can fix your brakes but you will have to wait until I have time later this afternoon."

Amit was baffled. He left the garage and drove to his office at school. A few minutes lapsed when he received a call. A woman was on the line. "Honey, do you want me to come over tonight? I can fix you a special meal."

"Who is this?" Amit asked.

"Very funny. Who do you think this is? Do you have another girl over there?"

Then Amit recognized the girl's voice. It was Angie. But how can that be? I haven't talked to her since she left school? "Ah, ah..., sure, ah..., okay, that would be great. Do you know where I live?" Amit said.

"I said, quit playing games Amit. I had a big day at the hospital." Angie was a registered nurse at a hospital near the school. "If you don't want me to come...."

"No, no, that would be great. I'll see you tonight," Amit said.

That evening after school, Amit rushed home. Was he dreaming or was Angie truly in his life? He went into his apartment and immediately noticed some changes inside. The room had different furniture and there were flowers on the table. There was a noticeable pleasant aroma in the apartment. He went to the bathroom and saw that someone else had left their toothbrush. In the shower, there were aromatic shampoos and conditioners. *These things are not mine. What is going on here?*

A half hour later, there was a jingling sound at the front door lock. Angie came into the apartment. She had her own key. She gave Amit a big kiss and asked him about his day. Amit fell into his chair astonished to see her. Her hair was longer and styled differently and she was a little older than he remembered. But she was more beautiful than ever. He could not figure out why or how she was there. Angie acted like they had been together for years. As promised, she cooked him dinner. Afterwards, they sat in the living room and Angie told him about her day. Amit wasn't hearing anything she said. He just stared at her in disbelief that she was in his apartment. Amit had not been with any women. When it was time for bed, they made love like it was their very first time. For Amit, perhaps it was.

Later that night, while she was lying next to him asleep, Amit tried to make sense of the change in events during the last 36 hours. After staying awake for most of the night, he concluded that his will had changed the course of history. By planting ideas into the minds of people he encountered, he could change their actions. More importantly, he could project his wishes onto people before they undertook some event, whether it was in the past or present time, thereby preventing the actions that were to come. Or at least the actions that he thought were to come. Through his mind implantation, *did I prevent Carl from raping Angie? Or was this current reality with Angie real and the rape imaginary? Was his previous memory a dream?* But his memories are so vivid. Amit was getting dizzy thinking about these various explanations. In the end, he was happy that he now had a life with the woman of his dreams and he did not tempt fate by trying to use his gift again. If he is able to change the future, he didn't want to risk losing his current reality.

Angie and Amit married later that year. Amit completed his doctoral degree and went on to complete a postdoctoral fellowship in clinical chemistry. Soon thereafter, he accepted a position as Assistant Professor of Pathology and Laboratory Medicine at the state's major medical school, and he was appointed as the Assistant Director of the Chemistry Laboratory at the University Hospital. Angie worked at the hospital as a registered nurse.

Amit enjoyed a productive career in clinical

laboratory science. He was the director of a lab that had a staff of 50 techs and produced millions of test results for patients seen at his hospital. He was also well funded to conduct research and publish his findings in peer-reviewed journals. His students loved his passion for the field and he trained many individuals who themselves went on to become laboratory directors. Perhaps his only disappointment was that he and Angie did not have any children. Angie died of an autoimmune disease when she was in her early 60s. Amit was distraught at the loss of his friend and lover. He was again alone in the world.

*

Many decades after his encounter with Carl in the auto shop, Amit began to think about how his life appeared to have changed that day. *Do I have the ability to change the will of people's intention? Can I implant seeds of doubt? More importantly, can I implant modern-day medical and laboratory knowledge that when acted upon, can change events?* Amit decided to tempt fate. He learned that through a "mind portal" he had access to, he could target a key scientist or doctor in history and that he had the ability to transplant an idea or suggestion without even seeing or meeting that individual. Once the seed has been planted, the individual would believe the idea was an original one. A little assistance from Amit would produce ripple effects that could change the modern world.

Amit was nearing 70 years of age. He had made his mark in the field and felt he now had a bigger calling. He has this talent that he did not dare to use before. But now that he was alone, he thought that his knowledge of laboratory medicine could influence important people in history and change the course of events for the better. He was willing to tempt his own reality for the sake of helping mankind in some manner....

*

Telepathy is a form of non-verbal communication whereby a person can transmit information to another without using any known physical or sensory interaction. The individual who has received the implant may not be aware of the transfer, and believes that he is the originator of that implant. There have been many science fiction movies about an individual who has telepathic powers. In the Star Wars *movies, many of the characters including Luke Skywalker and Obi-Wan Kenobi have telepathic powers that they use to alter the behavior of their enemies. The implanting of ideas may be an enhancement to telepathy. In the film,* In Your Eyes (2014), *takes telepathy one step further by enabling verbal communication between the two lovers who live far apart.*

The movie, Inception (2010) involves the use of telepathic powers for stealing corporate secrets. In science fiction definitions, inception means to instill an idea into another through dreams.

The concept of using telepathic powers to affect events that have already occurred in history has not been explored in the science fiction genre. An individual with this telepathic ability, coupled with today's knowledge, could produce fascinating changes in the course of human history.

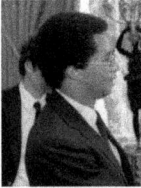

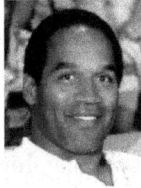

Ashwood

****

They had very different backgrounds. Chowder grew up in liberal San Francisco where his father was a well-known drag queen. Chowder's nickname was "Soup." As Soup's father divorced his wife when the boy was 5, he had little influence on his son's upbringing. Ashwood had been raised in conservative and racially segregated Richmond Virginia, the former capital of the Confederacy. His father had been a strict disciplinarian. Both men grew up to stand six foot one inches tall. But Soup was muscular and powerful. He was confident and brash and at one time was in a neighborhood gang. Ashwood was thin, slight of build, as such, his father forbade him to participate in football and so he chose tennis instead. He was reserved, thoughtful and highly intelligent. What they had in common was that both men were black, gifted athletes, and reached the pinnacle of their chosen sports.

Ashwood broke racial barriers during his rise in tennis. As a junior player, he was prohibited from playing in most of the regional tennis tournaments. At the time, there were no other prominent black male tennis professionals. There was only Althea Gibson who had excelled in women's tennis over a decade earlier. While most of the top players learned the game from country club tutors and coaches, Ashwood learned on the public courts of Richmond. When tennis talent was exhibited at an early age, Althea' coach, Walter Johnson, began to train young Ashwood. Within a few years, Ashwood won the National Indoor Junior Tennis Championship, and he received a scholarship to attend the University of California, Los Angeles.

Soup excelled in all sports, but particularly football as a youth. Because of the success of running back Jim Brown of the Cleveland Browns, Soup did not face the same level of discrimination that Ashwood confronted. Soup played two years at a junior college before joining University of Southern California on a football scholarship. During both years, Soup led the nation in rushing yardage among NCAA Division IA schools, and at the end of the season, he won College Football's most prestigious award. While both men attended schools in Southern California, Ashwood finished a year before Soup's arrival, and their paths did not cross.

Ashwood and Soup's professional careers were highly successful during the 10-plus years of their participation. Ashwood won Wimbledon, the U.S. Open, and the Australian Open championships and is still the only black male player to have done so. Soup led the NFL in rushing yardage on 4 occasions and was All Pro for 5 years.

His career rushing totals were second in the history of the game to that date.

Amit Savjani was a few years younger than either Ashwood or Soup. As a youth he was an avid sports fan and he followed the success of these two men on television. During the 1970s, there were only three major TV networks. With limited view options, tennis and football became highly popular, and Ashwood and Soup were among the first TV superstars of their sports. When they retired from competition, television network executives hired them as "color analysts" for broadcasts. At different times, both men worked alongside Sal Michaels, who was the "play-by-play" announcer. In the early 1980s, Ashwood and Soup met for the first time during an event hosted by Sal.

"My father wouldn't let me play football," Ashwood told Soup. "He thought it was a little too rough for a guy with my build. When I was small, they used to call me "bones.""

"I really envy you, Ashwood," Soup remarked. "I have this recurrent nightmare about this one line-backer from the Chicago Bears. His name was Butt Dickas. He would knock me out of bounds so hard that I would crash into the retaining wall and fall unconscious. I then wake up and realize that it was just a dream." Like most football players, but especially running backs, Soup had his share of concussions and traumatic brain injuries. While there was no such diagnosis at the time, it is highly likely that Soup suffered from post-traumatic stress disorder. "I get angry at my wife over the smallest most insignificant things. She is the love of my life, and I can't understand why I say nor do some of the things that I have done."

At the time of their meeting, Ashwood was nearing the end of writing a book on the history and difficulties of being an African American Athlete. He didn't want to tell Soup, but Ashwood himself had significant health issues. A few years earlier, he had suffered a heart attack and endured several cardiac surgeries to repair his ailing heart. A blood transfusion from his second heart surgery would ultimately lead to his premature mortality.

*

Amit took his students on ward rounds one day very early in his clinical chemistry career. They met an infectious disease doctor outside the room of one of his patients. "This man is suffering from an infection with pneumocystis pneumonia or "PCP." This man does not fit the pattern of a PCP infection, which is not common around here. There is something very different about this patient." This was Amit's first encounter with a patient who had AIDS, or acquired immune deficiency disorder. It would be a few more years before the human immunodeficiency virus or HIV would be discovered as the offending agent and the discovery of how AIDS was transmitted from one infected patient to another. As a blood-borne pathogen, HIV can be transmitted through transfusions of tainted blood. In 1985, the first laboratory test was approved by the FDA for diagnosis of AIDS. Soon thereafter, blood banks were testing donated units for the presence of antibodies to HIV. A mandate for testing of all donor blood units by blood banking laboratories lead to a great reduction in HIV cases.

Ashwood had been given blood as part of his open-heart surgery two years before the introduction of the HIV test and the testing of the blood supply for the presence of the virus. One of the units given to him was tainted by HIV, and Ashwood acquired the virus. Symptoms of AIDS became evident a few years later. After exhibiting some neurologic problems, tests revealed that he had *toxoplasmosis,* a common opportunistic infection among AIDS patients. An HIV test revealed that Ashwood had AIDS. He and his wife kept this information private for the next four years. When his declining physical appearance became evident, Ashwood revealed to the media that he acquired AIDS, and he died a year later of pneumonia brought on by his weakened medical condition.

Amit imagined how the world would be different had Ashwood lived. After retirement from tennis, Ashwood used his fame to support civil rights. He visited South Africa to protest against apartheid. He was arrested on several occasions for demonstrating in Washington DC. Ashwood was well respected among both the Caucasian and African American communities, and Amit believed his calming demeanour could defuse confrontational situations. Perhaps he could have been a mediator between sides as he had experienced both American social culture and the world of country clubs through his tennis success.

Through his mind portal, Amit convinced Ashwood to have his open-heart surgery performed at Stanford University Hospital in Palo Alto. Years before a laboratory test for HIV was implemented to screen blood products, the Blood Bank at Stanford was measuring CD4 and CD8 cells in donated blood. High numbers of CD4 white cells in blood help fight infection. CD8 white cells help kill cancer cells and other invaders. It was known that a low ratio of these circulating cells was characteristic of individuals infected with HIV, and these units were discarded. Stanford was ahead of other blood banks, which were not performing these tests in 1983. But at Stanford, use of this surrogate test prevented the HIV infection that Ashwood had acquired. Since Amit prevented the tennis star's HIV infection, Ashwood did not go on to establish an AIDS Foundation for educating people about HIV transmission, a negative consequence of Amit's portal suggestion. Instead, Ashwood continued to focus his attention towards domestic and international social issues.

*

In the initial real meeting with Soup, Ashwood was already infected with HIV. He knew his time was short and he wanted to devote it to his AIDS foundation. Now that history had been altered and that his blood was not infected, Ashwood became interested in Soup's plight of that of other football player's health issues. There were several prominent NFL players who suffered significant neurologic problems that we now know were likely due to concussions suffered while playing. Ashwood convinced Soup to work with him in studying the health and social history of other football players once they had retired from the game. They found that like Soup, many of these athletes had multiple divorces, complained of continuing health issues and had a high incidence of drug and alcohol abuse, and domestic violence.

"I am guilty of verbal and physical spousal abuse just as the other men we have interviewed," Soup confided. Ashwood knew all about it. Soup's wife placed multiple calls to 911 and to the Los Angeles Police Department because of her husband's attacks on her. Each time, the Officers would issue a warning but there were no arrests. After all, this was Soup, football hero and overall good guy. Sometimes the Officers would even ask for pictures with Soup and his autograph.

"I don't understand why I get into these rages, and I wish there was a way to control these impulses. At your suggestion, I regularly see a psychiatrist."

"Soup, I am here to help you in whatever way I can. I am going to give you the number to my personal long-range beeper. If you feel these negative urges, all you have to do is call me, and no matter where I am, or what I'm doing, I will get to a phone and get back to you. You have my promise."

Ashwood was true to his word. One day, Soup was visiting his young children from his second marriage. When he arrived at his former house, he saw that his ex-wife, Nicollette had spent the night with Donald, a young and highly attractive man. *That boy has to be 10 years younger than*

Nicollette. Soup started to clench his teeth and his hands formed a fist. He was seething. *How can she be with that boy with my children in the room next door? Is there no decency?* When Donald left the room, Soup and Nicollette had a heated argument.

"I forbid you to see that man. You are a bad influence on my children," Soup yelled.

"Your children?? I bore them and I alone am raising them now. We're not married anymore, remember? You have no right to tell me what I can do and can't do in my own fucking house. If you can't deal with this, then get out. Leave now!" Nicollette shouted, as she turned to leave the room.

Soup's emotions were totally out of control and he was not thinking rationally. He had a medium sized pocketknife attached to his car keys. He pulled them out and started slowly after Nicollette. *I'll fix them both. They are not going to make a fool out of me.* But as he pulled the blade out of his knife, a small piece of paper fell out. There was a telephone number written on the slip. Without Soup's knowledge, Ashwood had put it there thinking it might be important someday. Soup stopped, recognized that this was the number to Ashwood's beeper, and he sat down. He bent over and put his hands over his face. *Take a deep breath. What am I doing? Calm down. Ashwood is right, this is not me behaving in this way. I have a sickness. I need help.* Soup stood up, put his knife away, and headed for the front door.

Nicollete had called the police who arrived just as

Soup was stepping out. Soup put his hands up and stopped in this tracks. "Don't worry, guys. I'm leaving. Nicollette is safe and in the house with the kids."

The police could see that Soup was calm and that there were probably no issues. "Soup, we have to check this out. We need for you to stay with this officer," one of them said. When the other officer left, the remaining older policeman questioned Soup about the UCLA-USC football game that Soup had played in some decades earlier. The officer was just a teenage then and Soup was one of his heroes.

Nicollette and Donald were watching from the window and they both came outside. They could also see that Soup was no longer inflamed. The officers nevertheless went into the home and saw that the children were fine and playing in their room and there was no sign of any violence. The officer went back outside and told Soup he could leave. When he arrived back at his house, Soup beeped Ashwood who was in town. Ashwood came over to Soup's house and stayed over that night. They had a long talk about what could have happened. Overcome with emotions, Soup openly wept at what could have happened that night.

There were no more confrontations after that evening. Nicollette considered filing a restraining order but Donald convinced her not to do it. They married a few years later and Donald became a stepfather to Soup's children. Soup could see that Donald was a good man, and was very kind to Soup's kids.

*

In 1991, Rodney King, an African American male, was involved in a high-speed chase through the city of Los Angeles. When he stopped and got out of the car, police officers assaulted King. The incident was caught on film by a bystander. Four officers were tried and acquitted of criminal charges. This verdict led to riots in the city resulting in the deaths of 53 individuals. There was a tenuous relationship between the LA Police Department and African American citizens. Soup and Ashwood became strong advocates for the police department. With their sports celebrity status, they participated in community activities and education against prejudice. Through their efforts, the relationship of the police to minority groups gradually improved. The success of these programs spread to police departments in other cities.

The first case of HIV infection was thought to have occurred in 1959 in the Democratic Republic of the Congo. The first case in the U.S. occurred in 1981. The term "Acquired Immune Deficiency Disorder" was coined by the Centers for Disease Control a year later. The underlying etiology of AIDS was simultaneously discovered in 1984 by investigators at the Pasteur Institute, National Institute of Health, and the University of California, San Francisco. Within a year, a clinical laboratory test was developed that identified the presence of antibodies to the virus responsible for AIDS. Laboratory testing for CD4 (T helper) and CD8 (T killer) cells is performed today to evaluate the medical status of AIDS patients but they are not used for screening the donated blood supply. Today, there are newer assays, termed "HIV Combination Tests" that can detect the presence of tainted blood *earlier than the original assays launched in 1985.*

This is an alternate reality story about Arthur Ashe and Orenthal James ("O.J.") Simpson. Both highly successful athletes had a significant role in popular culture during their playing days and especially immediately after their retirement. Simpson made several Hollywood movies including the Naked Gun series while Ashe wrote articles for several magazines and newspapers and spent $300,000 of his own money to pen the three-part book, A Hard Road to Glory: A History of the African American Athlete. Simpson's conversion from athlete to a well-paid advertising icon, the earliest example for an African American athlete, is discussed in Ashe's "Since 1946" volume. OJ's endorsement success set the stage for other African American athletes to reach new financial heights, such as what was achieved by Tiger Woods.

As both men were broadcasters for their respective sports, they might have met through their mutual acquaintance with Al Michaels, who worked with both men at various times during the 1980s. The relationship between Ashe and Simpson is not documented, and their introduction through Michaels is fictitious. Given their similar accomplishments in sports, it is plausible that they could have become close friends and confidants.

Prior to Nicole Brown Simpson's divorce to OJ, there were several complaints filed by her with the local police regarding spousal abuse and domestic violence. The notion that Simpson suffered from chronic traumatic encephalopathy from concussions suffered as a running back is very possible but has not yet been documented. If OJ Simpson was responsible for the murders of Nicole and Ron Goldman, perhaps their deaths could have been avoided with the calming influence of Arthur Ashe. However, the international tennis star died of AIDS one year before Nicole's death.

The relationship between the police and minorities in America continues to be strained today. The recent events in Ferguson, Missouri, Baltimore, Maryland, and Dallas Texas attest to this fact. Part of the problem is the absence of an ambassador for peace, the role that Martin Luther King Jr. provided during the 1950s and 1960s. Perhaps if Arthur Ashe had avoided his HIV infection, he could have been this person, and our race relations might be better today.

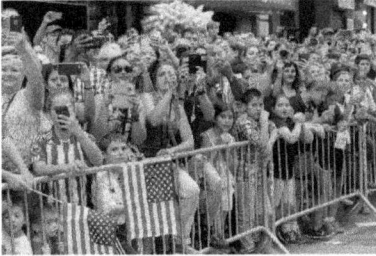

The Parade

****

Soup continued his life as a well-respected former star athlete. His agent was ambitious and pushed Soup into more and more commercial endorsements. As the national spokesman for the top rental car company, he will always be remembered as the guy who ran through airports jumping over baggage to get into his vehicle. Now, his face was on billboards and television commercials for many more products. He did ads for deodorants, soup, automobiles especially sports utility vehicles, Italian loafer shoes, and leather gloves. Because his body was as firm and muscular as it had been during his playing days, he appeared in a popular commercial modeling men's underwear. Soup's IMDb portfolio also continued to expand with more parts in Hollywood movies, television series, and talk shows. Soon, Soup became one of the most recognized faces in America of all time. Some considered his popularity to be as big as sports celebrities before him, including Arnold Palmer and Muhammad Ali, only to be surpassed by Tiger Woods a few year later. Soup worked for twenty years on the National Football League pregame shows. Based on his success as one of the best running backs in the history of the sport, his opinions about offensive schemes were valued by fans and coaches alike. He was a color analyst for Monday Night Football broadcasts alongside Al Michaels for five years.

Ashwood's life took a different course. He used his celebrity status to fight for equal rights among women, minorities, and the disenfranchised. He worked with Princess Diana to ban land mines. He helped raise tens of millions of dollars to help rebuild villages in Indonesia after the 2004 tsunami storm that killed hundreds of thousands of people. He helped Oprah Winfrey in her quest to educate African girls. He was a nominee for the 2009 Nobel Peace Prize that was awarded to Barack Obama. Ashwood was not disappointed that he didn't win, as he believed the President was more worthy of the award. In 2020, Ashwood was instrumental in curbing violent demonstrations during the "Black Lives Matter" protests. Soup and Ashwood continued to be friends and tried to meet whenever they were both in town.

*

Bob Walker grew up in San Francisco and graduated from Galileo High School precisely ten years after Soup. As an avid football fan, Bob tracked Soup's outstanding college and professional career. Although he was on the school's football team, Bob knew his calling would be medicine so after getting a bachelor's degree in biology from the University of California, Berkeley, he went to UC San Francisco for medical school. When he received his medical degree, he took his residency and fellowship at the Massachusetts General Hospital in Boston. After completing these programs, Bob stayed in Boston in the Department of Medicine at Beth Israel. Then one day after serving 6 years on the faculty, he told his wife, Francie, a nurse and lifelong New Englander, that he wanted to move their young family to San Francisco.

"Boston was great for my career and the kids have done well here, but it's time for us to return to my home back in California. Besides, the Patriots' stink and I'm missing out on seeing all of the 49ers teams." Little did he know then that Tom Brady who grew up in nearby San Mateo would soon arrive and the Patriots would become the dominant team in the sport. Reluctant at first, Francie did agree to move. The children were still young and became excited about moving to the Golden State. They knew the lifestyle there having visited San Francisco every summer to see their grandparents. Bob had no trouble landing a position as a hospital physician at UCSF's Moffett Long Hospital and became an Associate Professor of Medicine. Bob moved up the ranks and within 20 years, he became Chief of the Department. Bob became a season ticket holder for the San Francisco 49ers and watched many games at Candlestick Park. When the 49ers moved to Levi Stadium in neighboring Santa Clara, Bob maintained his seat license with the team. Over the years, his seat location improved, and he was now on row 30 near midfield.

*

After their last Super Bowl win, the San Francisco 49ers entered several decades of decline. Head coaches and players came and went. None during this era had the star power of Joe Montana, Steve Young, Jerry Rice and Ronnie Lott. The team did have a brief resurgence when Jim Harbaugh was hired away from Stanford to be the head coach. They reached Super Bowl LXVII after the 2013 season, but the 49ers lost to the Baltimore Ravens coached by Jim's older brother, John (that Super Bowl was nicknamed the "Harbaugh Bowl"). Soon thereafter, Jim left for the University of Michigan and the team faced several more lean years. That all changed when the team owners hired John Lynch as General Manager and Kyle Shanahan as the head coach. Lynch played 15 years in the NFL with the Tampa Bay Buccaneers and Denver Broncos. When he retired in 2008, John consulted with Soup about a career in broadcasting. Six days after announcing his retirement, he joined the Fox Television Studio broadcast team as a color analyst.

Kyle, the son of a former NFL head coach, was an assistant coach for several teams before becoming head coach of the 49ers. He was the offensive coordinators for the Atlanta Falcons that lost the game to the Patriots after having a having a 28 to 3 lead. John Lynch convinced Kyle to hire

Soup as a special consultant for the team's offense. Soup worked with the 49ers collection of talented but unheralded running backs. Shanahan's first two years with the team were mired with injuries to several of his key players and they had a losing record. Then in 2019, the team make a remarkable break through by winning their first 8 games of that season, and 12 of their first 13. They accomplished this by running the football. The team was second in the league in rushing yards gained per game. The 49ers easily won their first two games of the playoffs, again by gaining yards on the ground instead of through the air. The team earned a trip to the Super Bowl LIV in Miami against the American Football Conference winner, the Kansas City Chiefs. The game was close, but the 49ers held a 10-point lead mid-way through the fourth quarter. Then the opposing team behind their star quarterback, Patrick Mahomes took the lead with two late fourth quarter touchdowns. Fans began to think about the game the Falcons lost under Shanahan's offense. The 49ers had still had a chance with just over two minutes left. During the two-minute warning, Soup, who had a bird's eye view from the coach's box upstairs, and was able to get a brief word to Shanahan through his headphone.

"Coach, they are looking for mid-range passes and are covering Kittle and Sanders like a blanket." Kittle and Sanders were among the team's leading receivers. "If we score too soon with a long pass, it will give Mahomes time to mount a game winning score. Let's cram it down their throats with our running game. From up here, we can see that their linebackers are gassed. This plan has worked all year." Shanahan agreed and changed his strategy. He called for a series of runs, keeping full back Kyle Juszczyk in the backfield blocking. They ran a sweep to Raheem Mostert for 12 yards, then a handoff up the middle to Tevin Coleman. Jimmy Garoppolo picked up 8 more yards on a quarterback draw. Then Mostert got the ball again on a reverse pitch. The touchdown was an end around play to Deebo Samuel. George Kittle, as he had done all year, made the key block. With the extra point, the 49ers were ahead 27 to 24. More importantly, they left Mahomes and the Chiefs only 15 seconds left. This was not enough time for Mahomes to score, and the 49ers celebrated their 6th Superbowl win in 24 years.

*

On that Super Bowl Sunday, Dr. Bob Walker assembled his team of doctors and nurses in the UCSF Department of Medicine conference room to initiate the COVID-19 Command Center.

"I really want to thank each and every one of you for coming in this afternoon and giving up your Sunday. I want to impress on you the seriousness of the pandemic occurring in China," Dr. Walker said.

Dr. Arun Seagal was head of this Command Center. "We have what appears to be two cases of COVID-19 infection now in the Bay Area. One in San Benito County and another from this morning in Santa Clara. This could get real serious here and we must prepared for the worse."

The individuals attending the meeting left the room with specific orders. The team needed to know how many emergency departments beds were available at the various UCSF hospitals, and the daily census of admission. The number of intensive care unit beds available was also determined. An inventory of personal protective equipment was made. The schedule of elective surgeries and procedures was mapped. "Someone needs to contact the CDC to see if there are any virus tests available now to confirm a COVID-19 infection."

On Monday, the first of many thousands of individuals would arrive at hospitals in San Francisco suspected of being infected with COVID-19.

*

At the headquarters of the San Francisco 49ers, the event group were talking with San Francisco city officials about hosting a parade through the streets, cumulating with speeches by players and coaches at City Hall. The Bay Area hosted six championship celebrations over the past 10 years, three each for the San Francisco Giants baseball team and the Golden State Warriors basketball team. As American cities go, only Boston has enjoyed more championships in recent years (with the Patriots, Red Sox, Celtics and Bruins).

"We want this to be special because it has been 24 years since our last championship," the head of marketing said to the group. The parade was scheduled for the Wednesday after the Super Bowl game. The mayor's office was involved with the planning. Like the Giant's parade, it would start at near the century old Ferry Building and traverse down Market Street to City Hall. Nobody at the time was thinking that this was a bad idea.

The weather was warm and there was no rain. Nearly two million people crammed the streets of San Francisco. Everybody was in close contact with each other trying to get a glimpse of their Super Bowl heroes. There were a few individuals attended who were unknowingly infected with COVID but showed no symptoms. By coughing, yelling and cheering, they infected dozens of others in attendance. Then these individuals went home and began infecting their loved ones. Within a week, all of the San Francisco Hospitals were inundated with COVID-infected patients. The death rate began to mount. There were shortages of laboratory tests for detecting the virus and supplies such as nasal swabs. N95 masks were in short supply and not available to all of the healthcare workers that needed them. Soon, some of the people on the frontline became infected. With a surge of ICU patients, ventilators became in short demand. The UCSF Command Center did what it could to alleviate these shortages. The committee made a plea to other communities that had not yet been infected. But they could not keep up with the demand.

In hindsight, Amit could see that parade was responsible for escalating the rate of COVID-infection, and that the team Super Bowl victory was a defeat for the Bay Area. He knew he had the power to do something and he acted. The role that Soup had in saving the game for the

49ers was well documented by interviews with Coach Shanahan. Unfortunately, Soup himself became infected while attending the parade, and was among the first to be admitted to UCSF. Now in his seventies, Soup overweight and had type 2 diabetes. He had difficulty breathing so he was admitted to the intensive care unit on a ventilator. Fighting off linebackers was nothing compared to this battle. He was treated with various medications include hydroxychloroquine and anti-inflammatory agents, and at first, it appeared to help. But his illness relapsed on the next day, and he died a few days later. Football fans across the country mourned for the death of their fallen star. An in-person memorial was not permitted.

Amit went into Mind Portal and targeted Soup during the Super Bowl, in order to change the existing reality. At the critical two-minute warning of the fourth quarter, he planted the notion that Soup should not call Kyle Shanahan at this critical junction. *The man is a genius when it comes to offense. His schemes during the past year got us to this point. Trust that he will make the right decisions and we'll win the game.* The re-written history showed that on the next play, Jimmy Garopollo overthrew Sanders who was open down field. On fourth down, Jimmy got tackled behind the line of scrimmage and the ball was turned over on downs to the Chiefs. They scored a meaningless touchdown that padded the lead and won the game. Afterwards, Soup was upset with himself that he didn't make that call to the coach. Instead of San Francisco, the Chiefs hosted a victory parade in their hometown on that following Wednesday. But unlike San Francisco, Kansas City was yet to have their first COVID-19 case. Therefore, the parade did not become a source of infection to Missourians. Back in San Francisco, the COVID infection rate was modest in the absence of the parade. It never reached the level of other California cities such as Santa Clara and Los Angeles Counties, or close to the tragic pandemic that occurred in New York City. Through his mind portal, Amit save hundreds of lives in the Bay.

Soup survived the infection and made public infomercials to tell citizens of the importance of staying home. He sold his 1968 Heisman trophy award for $800,000 to a collector and donated the money to help families of COVID-19 victims in Santa Clara. While Soup survived the infection, his friend Ashwood, who was working in South America at the time, was one of the early victims. His pre-existing coronary heart disease was a contributing factor. Drs. Segal, Walker, and the all of the UCSF COVID-19 Command Center remained busy providing the resources, medical advice, and statistics for the many cases they saw.

*

On March 16, San Francisco Mayor London Breed issued a shelter-in-place mandate for the city and county. Four days later, California Governor Gavin Newsom ordered it for the entire state. They were the first city and state in the U.S. to do so. It would be another 11 days before President Donald Trump mandated it for the rest of the nation. Afterwards, life in the United States and throughout the world changed dramatically. The stock market suffered unprecedented losses. Unemployment skyrocketed. There was much opposition to shut down by the nation. Critics point out that there are hundreds of thousands of deaths each year due to infections by influenza. However, in the absence of a vaccine and effective therapies, political leaders were convinced that more drastic measures to contain SARS-CoV-2 was warranted.

On March 18, Governor Gavin Newsom sent a letter to the President stating that 56% or 25.5 million California residents will be infected with COVID-19. Based on these projections, Drs. Niraj Sehgal and Bob Wachter continued to prepare UCSF hospitals for the worse. Fortunately, these surge estimates did not occur in the city in those early months.

The decision to essentially quarantine most of the California population in March 2020 was heralded as the main reason why infections in California did not reach the heights of the East Coast. Unfortunately, during the fall and winter months of 2020, the subsequent opening of the state's businesses may have led to higher rates of infections in California than elsewhere. The Bay Area, however, had a lower rate of infections and deaths in the 2021 surge than elsewhere in the State.

Tom Brady would lead a second NFL team, the Tampa Bay Buccaneers to the Super Bowl (his 10th overall) and his 7th overall victory. He is really the GOAT (Greatest Of All Time).

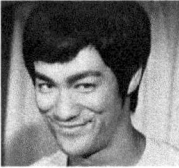

Asian Lives Matter

****

Amit Savjani's boyhood hero was the martial arts extraordinaire and actor, Bruce Lee. Smaller than the other boys, Amit tried to imagine how he could fend off the local boys who regularly harassed him. Lee's father was a Hong Kong opera star and was on tour with his wife in 1960 when Bruce was born in San Francisco's Chinatown district. In Chinese horoscope, this was the year of the Dragon. His mother was part English. At three months of age, Bruce's family moved back to Hong Kong where he was raised. As a teenager, Bruce Lee was involved in many fights. His father enrolled him into a martial arts school where he learned Gung Fu. Because the boy continued to get into fights with rival students and gang members, his father decided to send him to the United States. He first lived in San Francisco to stay with his older sister and later moved to Seattle, Washington.

Amit watched the television show, *The Green Hornet*, where Lee played the part of Kato. In previous television and cinematic productions, Asians were cast as being weak, submissive, and cartoon-like in their appearance and dialogue. Kato was a strong and confident character which initiated the breakdown of this stereotype. While Kato had only s few lines within the show's weekly script, Lee's martial arts prowess showed that Asians can assume dominant masculine roles. Unfortunately, America was not ready for Asians as leading men and *The Green Hornet* was cancelled after just one season and 26 episodes.

As a pre-teenager, Amit tried to emulate his hero. He started to exercise more and lifted weights. In front of a full-length mirror, he started to shadow kick and punch like Bruce Lee did. He wanted to join a karate gym, but his mother did not approve. Amit went on his own to the gym to purchase a set of numchucks. These were two wooden sticks attached to each other by a chain. Lee trained with numchucks by rapidly whipping them around his head, neck, arms, and shoulders. Amit was clumsy as a child, not a gifted athlete like Bruce Lee. Even by starting out very slowly, he banged his head with numchucks several times leaving visible bumps and bruises. He began to wear wool hats in class that further separated him from his classmates. Amit's mother saw the marks on his head and thought that her son was getting into fights. Amit told her that they were self-inflected by use of the training sticks.

"How could you be so stupid?" she asked. "For a smart kid you really are a dumb-chuck."

"Yeah, I know mom," Amit said. *What was I thinking? I could never be Bruce Lee. But I'm still going to follow him,"* Amit thought.

His mother confiscated the sticks and they soon became dumpster-chucks. Amit agreed that he wasn't meant for that type of training and resumed focus on his schoolwork.

Bruce Lee appeared in a few episodes of other television shows after *Green Hornet*, but his acting career was largely at a standstill. The Hollywood producer Fred Weintraub suggested to Lee that he move back to Hong Kong. Lee was unaware that his Kato character on *The Green Hornet* was widely popular in Hong Kong, and that he was already recognized by town residents as a star. Bruce Lee signed a film contract with Golden Harvest, a local movie studio to star in two feature length movies that highlighted his martial arts skills. The success of these films led to the production of two others. One was made in 1972 that included a fight scene with Chuck Norris, which helped launched Norris' own martial arts movie career. The other was completed in 1973 that included the NBA Hall of Famer, Kareen Abdul-Jabbar, who was in the 3rd of his 20 NBA seasons. During the filming of this last movie, *Enter the Dragon*, the American studio Warner Brothers became part of the production. Having been a fan of Lee's Kato character, it was natural that Amit would be a big fan of his movies and he watched them multiple times. It was a particularly sad day for him when Bruce Lee suddenly died on July 20, 1973 at the age of 32.

*

Amit went on to become a clinical laboratory director of a major academic medical center. Amit was one of the key healthcare workers dealing with the deadly COVID-19 pandemic. He, his colleagues, and staff were on the frontline providing testing for the virus as well as assessing a patient's immune response with antibody testing. While not trained as a microbiologist, Amit had to shift his focus from clinical chemistry and toxicology to handle the testing for this infectious disease. The State of California, and the country as a whole were placed on lockdown in the Spring of 2020. Only essential workers were permitted to leave their homes. Since testing for the presence of the virus was essential for determining who was infected and required medical attention, Amit came into the clinical laboratory and office working every day. If fighting the country's worst pandemic since the 1918 Spanish Flu was not enough, the deaths of George Floyd, Breonna Taylor, and others provided even more stress to an already traumatized nation. As a son of immigrants, Amit faced some discrimination as a child and as an adult. The deaths of Floyd and Taylor prompted Amit to study racism against Asians in America.

*

After the California Gold Rush in 1849, Chinese immigrants came to the U.S. to work in the gold mines, garment industry, in the agricultural fields, and building the transcontinental railroad. Many worked harder than their white counterparts and accepted lower wages. This led to considerable resentment by the Caucasian population. In 1871 in Los Angeles, an argument over a prostitute resulted in the accidental shooting of a white civilian, who came to the aid of policemen. This led to a riot where a mob of 500 angry white people who shot, hung, and stabbed 18 Chinese men to death. Only one of the victims was involved with the shooting. A year later, 9 men involved with the mob killings were convicted of manslaughter, but all were released by the California Supreme Court a year later.

Continued tensions between whites and Chinese on the West Coast led the U.S. Congress to introduce legislation to limit the number of Chinese that could legally enter the U.S. In 1882, The Chinese Exclusion Act was passed which suspended the immigration of Chinese laborers into the U.S. for 10 years and prohibited them from citizenship. It was the first time that the U.S. placed broad restrictions on immigration. After the Act was expired, it was extended for another decade and expanded to include Hawaii and the Philippines. In 1902, Congress made the Exclusion Act indefinite. It was not repealed until 1943 through the Magnuson Act, when China became an ally to the Americans during World War II. It was a token gesture by the Roosevelt administration to appease their ally. Only 105 visas per year were granted. One year before Magnuson Act, Japanese citizens on the West Coast were subjected to internment camps.

The discrimination against Asians has occurred

throughout the history of the United States. These acts are not as well publicized today as the discrimination observed against Jews, Blacks, and Muslims. That changed with the onset of the coronavirus outbreak. On January 28, 2021, Vicha Ratanapakdee an 84-year old immigrant was pushed to the ground and died of a brain hemorrhage. On March 16, 2021, 8 people were killed by gunshot in an Atlanta spa. Six of these victims were Asian women. While it is not clear if these deaths from the spa were related to an anti-Asian hate crime, it has recently spurred hundreds of others throughout the U.S. to attack Asians. Amit was particularly distressed that these attacks occurred within his own neighborhood in San Francisco where he lives and works. He wondered if he could reverse this situation using his Mind Portal.

*

The cause of Bruce Lee's death has been debated for over 40 years. The actor collapsed on the set in May of 1973. Doctors diagnosed him as having cerebral edema, i.e., water around the brain. It was a very hot day in Hong Kong. In the studio, the air conditioning was turned off as it was added background noise. Two months later, Lee had another lapse into unconsciousness while visiting the home of a fellow actor. He was sent by ambulance to a hospital, but he was dead on arrival. An autopsy again showed brain swelling. A few months before Lee's first episode, he had his sweat glands removed from his arm pits. As with any finely tuned athlete, sweating is a major means to dissipate heat generated by strenuous exercise. As an actor playing a role, excessive perspiration produces unsightly stains requiring bathing and wardrobe changes. Lee felt that the removal of these glands would help the production team to stay on time and on budget. Physicians and biographers have suggested that heat stroke may have been the precipitating event in causing Lee's death. Amit recalled his own experiences reviewing clinical lab test results on patients suffering from excessive heat.

*

On September 1, 2017, high atmospheric pressure occurred over Northern California producing a heat wave. A temperature of 106 degrees occurred in San Francisco, breaking the previous record of 103. Unlike the inland valley areas where triple digit temperatures are common, residents of San Francisco rarely see hot temperatures as the marine layer keeps the conditions cooler. Many houses do not have or need air conditioning. On this particular weekend, dozens of individuals came to the emergency department at the General with heat stroke due to excessive temperature exposure. Amit noted that these patients had abnormal lab results for blood gases and electrolytes, essential for maintaining a healthy homeostasis. Certain organs are particularly vulnerable to hyperthermia including the heart and liver. A breakdown of skeletal muscles leads to kidney failure if untreated. Reducing body temperature with compresses and ice baths, and regulation of circulating electrolyte concentrations is essential for survival. As a toxicologist, Amit also reviewed medico-legal cases of individuals who died of heat stroke while attending outdoor music events. These rave festivals are often held in the desert during the hot summer months. There is a lot of dancing that takes place during the concerts that further accelerates body temperatures. Amit's own clinical research lab showed that the use of Ecstasy inhibits the body's natural thermo regulation and puts users at additional risks for hyperthermia.

Amit wondered how the world would be different had Bruce Lee survived his heat stroke. The key was Lee's decision to remove his sweat glands. Amit entered his mind portal and implanted an idea directly into actor's mind and reversed the actor's decision to have this surgery. *Sweating is necessary to keep cool. You are Bruce Lee. You are the best martial arts performer on the planet. Why do you care what anybody thinks? That never bothered you before. Does anybody believe that you wouldn't sweat?*

That brain implant changed everything. Lee canceled his surgery with his dermatologist. As a result, he did not suffer any collapses in 1973. Instead, for the next 10 years, Lee made dozens of more martial-arts style feature-length movies. After *Enter the Dragon*, he completed *Game of Death*, planned at the time of his original death. His films evolved when he asked screenwriters to add humor to his dialogue and fighting sequences. In the original history, Jackie Chan became a popular star after Lee's death, and used comedic scenes that entertained audiences for decades.

In the late 1980s and early 1990s, Bruce Lee now entering his fifties, received leading roles in romantic, and dramatic films that led him away from his Gung Fu upbringing. As a movie star, Bruce was as just as famous as another former world class athlete, Arnold Schwarzenegger. They alternated in producing box-office hits. When his son Brandon became an actor, Bruce was there to mentor him. Brandon was accidently shot and killed on the set of a movie in 1993, however this did not occur with his father's survival.

*

In the year 2003, the citizens of California were unhappy with the actions of Governor Gray Davis, and a recall election was held. Arnold Schwarzenegger and Bruce Lee were the top candidates. The body builder turned actor defeated the Gung Fu turned actor. Schwarzenegger served two terms and was succeeded in by the former Governor Jerry Brown. Gavin Newsom, Mayor of San Francisco, became the Lieutenant Governor. Upon Newsom's resignation, Edwin Lee, the City Administrator, was appointed by the Board of Supervisors to serve out Newsom's remaining 1-year term in 2011. In the fall of 2011, the city held an election for the permanent mayor. Bruce Lee decided to run against Edwin. Coincidently both men lived in Seattle when they were younger but didn't know each other. During the locally publicized debate, the two Lees highlighted their different platform. Edwin stressed the importance of revitalizing business and commerce while his opponent was against gun violence and crimes based on race, religion, and sexual orientation. Bruce Lee defeated Edwin in the election and took office in 2012.

In the real history, Edwin Lee was the San Francisco Mayor until he unexpectedly died of a sudden heart attack in December 2017. Dealing with the COVID-19 pandemic was left to his successor, London Breed, who under her brilliant leadership, San Francisco experienced the lowest rate of infection and death of any major U.S. city. Without the stress of the mayor's office, the election of Bruce Lee would have resulted in Edwin Lee's avoidance of his fatal heart attack.

Once in office, Bruce Lee invested heavily in law enforcement. As someone who experienced discrimination, he set up a mandatory training program for police officers to receive diversity training. He hired minorities into key supervisory positions. He asked the city's district attorney to aggressively prosecute individuals who committed hate crimes. Through his Hollywood connections, he produced local public service announcements promoting anti-racism. To complement the social media campaign, "Black Lives Matter," which began in 2013, Lee initiated the "Asian Lives Matter" movement within the city that received national attention. In public appearances, Lee promoted the phrase, "a kinder and gentler America," one that was coined by President George H.W. Bush during his presidency decades earlier. He served for one term and retired in 2016 at the age of 76 and was succeeded by London Breed.

Amit could see that by enabling Bruce Lee to survive, hate crimes, senseless shooting, and the overall mental health in America improved. Who would have thought that the avoidance of a simple surgical procedure could have this impact?

*

Sweat is caused by the eccrine gland found in all areas of the body but are concentrated in the hands and feet. During heavy exercise, a person can lose 1-4 liters of fluid per hour. Apocrine gland found in the armpits and perianal area. Body odor, also known as osmidrosis, occurs when skin bacteria is mixed with sweat. The number of sweat glands found in the axillary areas of the body is determined by the ATP-binding cassette transporter, a protein that exports substances from cells. In humans, there are two major genetic variances. The G allele is dominant while the A allele is recessive. This means that individuals with one or two G alleles have a phenotype associated with underarm odor. Individuals from Korea, China, Mongolia and western Japan have the recessive A allele, whereas most Caucasians have the G allele. Interestingly, this gene also dictates whether a person's ear wax is wet (dominant genotype) or dry (recessive genotype). Some believe that dry wax is protective against ear infections. As Bruce Lee's mother was part Caucasian, it is possible that the actor inherited one G allele from her and suffered from hyperhidrosis, excess sweat. Therefore, he felt the need to remove these glands through surgical resection. Today, there are other ways besides resection, including laser treatment, liposuction, curettage (scraping) and cutting the nerve that feeds the gland.

Prior to becoming a television and movie star, Bruce Lee operated and taught at martial arts schools. Many of the schools in Hong Kong at that time discriminated against individuals who were not 100% Chinese. Lee embraced all races and ancestries in his instruction. He married Linda Emery, one of his gung fu students, and their two children Brandon and Shannon are admixed. Bruce Lee's philosophy stressed peace and harmony, with an emphasis on self-control, to strive for the best in life, and have respect for others. Linda and Shannon have continued Lee's teaching for nearly 50 years after Lee's death.

Crimes against Asians and Pacific Islanders in America have been on the rise since the onset of the SARS-CoV-2 pandemic. To some extent, it was fueled by some politicians who labeled the outbreak in speeches and social media as the "China Virus" and "Kung Flu." While it is true that the cases occurred in Wuhan, China, this label suggests to some uninformed individuals that the virus was created by the Chinese government. How this version of the coronavirus was created is unknown. There is no credible evidence to date, however, that it was man-made, and there are no documents that any government purposefully created this killer. Other pandemics have been labeled according to where the initial cases were identified. The H1N1 influenza pandemic lasted from 1918 to 1920 and killed 500 million people was known as the "Spanish flu." At that time, there was no political motivation to label this deadly virus as such. Today, placing blame is a strategy to deflect inadequacies of governmental policies. Since the very beginning of the outbreak, international health organizations such as written by the WHO have warned against the practice of linking a virus to a location or ancestry. An issue for some Asians, particularly elderly ones, is the reluctance to disclose a violent act that they may have suffered for fear of retribution.

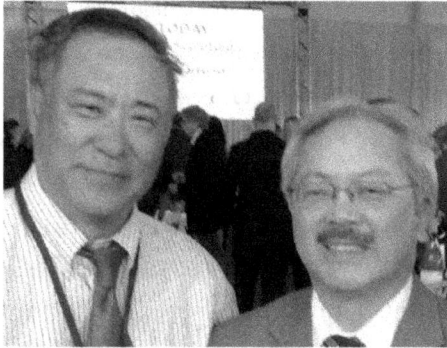

Epilogue

****

Not since the Civil War have our nation been so divided as they were in the year 2020. The political divisions between liberal democrats and conservative Republicans have been striking. Some of this disparity is over racial inequalities, highlighted with the deaths of George Floyd and Breonna Taylor at the hands of the local police.

The COVID-19 pandemic has served to further highlight these differences. Elderly populations are more vulnerable than the young. Individuals with co-morbidities are at greater risk than healthy individuals. Minorities especially Latina and African Americans are more vulnerable than Caucasians. Men have higher infection rates than women. Asian Americans are being discriminated by some who blame their ancestors from China for the outbreak. This may be a sequel to the discrimination of Islamic American citizens that occurred after the 9/11 attack.

SARS-CoV-2 has further widened the gap between the rich from the poor. It could be stated that workers in the high-technical industry have actually benefited from COVID-19, in that they can continue their jobs by working at home. This is leading to a migration of high-cost living accommodations close to tech headquarters to lower housing further away. Blue-collar employees are associated with lower incomes and cannot stay home to earn a living. For those who are able to work, they are risking their lives and those of their immediate families. Unemployment in these sections are high, leading to unprecedented homelessness within our communities.

There is also an educational divide between wealth and poor populations. Students are not able to attend classes and are given instructions virtually. Families that can afford home computers and fast internet services are advantaged relative to children from underprivileged families who do not have these resources. If the pandemic is prolonged, these students will not be able to compete for the higher paying jobs furthering the divide.

During these difficult times, I found it important to provide both informational content on COVID-19 and some entertainment and even humor. Adding levity to a dire situation has been done before. Through the various conflicts of the 20th century, Bob Hope provide our troops stationed overseas a break from the rigors of combat. I was hoping to fulfill a similar purpose with this book.

I am humbly aware that millions of people have died worldwide from COVID19 and acknowledge that we are in a very serious situation. My sincere apologies to anyone who found this book to be inappropriate or distasteful. This was certainly not my intent. My goal was to use a little levity instead, to relieve the persistently and relentless stress and anxiety of this pandemic. I hope I have achieved this goal and you have enjoyed this book.

It was not my intent to provide political commentary to the events that led up to the Presidential Elections of 2020. I attempted to relay the facts as I saw and read them, recognizing that there are biases from writers, newscasters and newspapers.

Images courtesy of Wikimedia Commons and Dreamstime.

Epilogue

www.ingramcontent.com/pod-product-compliance
Lightning Source LLC
Chambersburg PA
CBHW062051270326
41931CB00013B/3023